Women's Perspectives on the Solution Focused Approach

W0113604

This book is a distinctive collection of narratives of female Solution Focused practitioners, from across six continents, sharing their unique ways of using the approach at personal, professional, and social levels.

Nineteen female practitioners from around the world share their practice and experience, and reflect on how their gender has influenced their work within different cultural, sociological, and socio-economic contexts. The editors introduce the concepts of a Solution Focused DNA and then encourage the contributors as well as the readers to answer questions such as: What are the common characteristics that are a part of your Solution Focused DNA? Which of them are related to gender, which of them to the Solution Focused Approach, and which of them to your sociocultural context? Contributors also provide insights on how they work from the Solution Focused approach integrating their own creative styles using embodiment and dance, animal assisted therapy, and humour. The chapters in this book explore a wide variety of themes and contexts, including shelters, trauma, the LGBTQ community, prisons, schools, refugee camps, veterans, the medical field, research, children, and more.

This book will inspire practitioners regardless of gender to reflect on their own practice and to use and apply the Solution Focused Approach in innovative and creative ways.

Anne-Marie Wulf is a social worker and family therapist who lives and works in Copenhagen, Denmark. She's the director of the Danish Solution Focused Institute and the current president of the European Brief Therapy Association (EBTA). She has authored and contributed to several books on the Solution Focused approach.

Jacqui von Cziffra-Bergs is a practising psychologist from Johannesburg, South Africa, and the director of the Solution Focused Institute of South Africa. She was an associate professor at the University of Johannesburg and has written five books on the Solution Focused approach.

Women's Perspectives on the Solution Focused Approach

International Applications and Interventions

Edited by Anne-Marie Wulf and Jacqui von Cziffra-Bergs

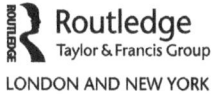

Routledge
Taylor & Francis Group

LONDON AND NEW YORK

Designed cover image: © Whackdesign

First edition published 2025
by Routledge
4 Park Square, Milton Park, Abingdon, Oxon, OX14 4RN

and by Routledge
605 Third Avenue, New York, NY 10158

Routledge is an imprint of the Taylor & Francis Group, an informa business

British Library Cataloguing-in-Publication Data
A catalogue record for this book is available from the British Library

ISBN: 9781032553481 (hbk)
ISBN: 9781032553474 (pbk)
ISBN: 9781003430254 (ebk)

DOI: 10.4324/9781003430254

Typeset in Times New Roman
by Newgen Publishing UK

In loving memory of
Insoo Kim Berg
(1934 – 2007)
- the greatest Solution Focused
female voice ever

Contents

Foreword by Eve Lipchik

Typical of thoughtful women, when Anne-Marie and Jacqui asked me whether I would be willing to write a foreword for this book they assured me that given my advanced years it could be brief. Little did they know that the minute I started to read this book it would draw me in to the extent that it was hard to put down. However, something occurred to me as I was reading. I wondered whether all these wonderful Solution Focused therapists all over the world knew about how it all started and the significance of women in that process. So, I thought I would describe that briefly.

In the mid-1970s Insoo Berg and Steve de Shazer, a married couple, became intrigued with a model called "Brief Therapy" developed at the Mental Research Institute in Palo Alto, California by Paul Watzlawick, John Weak*lland, and Richard Fisch. They decided to attempt to develop a similar but more systemic approach and to call it "Brief Family Therapy". For that purpose, they established the Brief Family Therapy Center in Milwaukee and were joined by Jim Derks, Elam Nunnally, Marilyn LaCourt, and me in 1978. We started out with just one interviewing room that had a one-way mirror, behind which we observed sessions when clients gave written permission.

In the early 1980s a dramatic change occurred because of the experimental way we often worked. One day at the end of a family session someone behind the mirror suggested that we change the usual first session "homework" assignment. "Instead of asking them to report next week what else they want to change in the family, let's ask them to report what they DON'T want to change!" In the next session the family reported many things that had gone well that week instead of complaining about the problems. This was different, so we tried it again and again, and that is how the Solution Focused approach was born.

Gender equality was never an issue at the Brief Family Therapy Center even though it was, and still is, one in the United States that needs much improvement. However, it cannot be compared to the conditions women have to live with in some of the countries represented by contributors to this book. The styles of the Brief Family Therapy group members clearly differed. There is no question that Insoo, Marilyn, and I were more conversational and warm with clients than the men were. Steve was famous throughout his career for his minimalist style that consisted of rarely having eye contact with clients. Jim and Elam did less "socialising" and got to the point much sooner. The continuing work and creativity of many of the past students and visitors, women being prominent among them, is responsible for making the Solution Focused approach the now universally appreciated therapeutic modality it has become.

Now to the book! Once I started to read it, I could not put it down until I had read every word. I was very impressed with the concept. The structure itself, multi-layered conversations, is brilliant. In each chapter the specific author first talks about her history and work; then Anne-Marie poses a series of questions, including one about an exercise the author uses in her work; this is concluded with a discussion between her and Jacqui. Their discussion expands on and reinforces the material previously covered, and then, when appropriate, links it with related material of other authors in the book. An extra-charming and creative touch is that Anne-Marie and Jacqui's comments are identified by a different female emoji. The sum total of all these chapters results in a tapestry of Solution Focused thinking that leads to a deeper and broader understanding of its practice, and one that has the means to offer a learning experience for beginners as well as the most seasoned Solution Focused therapist.

The cultural diversity of the contributors and their varied professional back-grounds offer a multifaceted perspective of the practice of Solution Focused Therapy of seasoned therapists, as well as some new to the practice. The variety of creative applications of the theoretical foundation of approach is impressive and often very illuminating. While some therapists are quite faithful in applying it as written and taught, others show amazing creativity in adapting it to fit their culture, the problem they are dealing with, or the setting in which they apply it. I cannot remember reading any book about Solution Focused therapy that has offered as many perspectives on the application of Solution Focused therapy as this one.

Women's Perspectives on the Solution Focused Approach: International Applications and Interventions is a very valuable contribution to the Solution Focused literature. I have no doubt that this book will broaden the perspective of all readers and that they will feel enriched much more than they expected.

Eve Lipchik
September 2023

Foreword by Yvonne Dolan

It was a great pleasure to read the various chapters of this book describing the unique ways that each of these inspiring women has incorporated the Solution Focused approach into her work. And it was wonderful to read the written exchanges between Anne-Marie and Jacqui as they responded to one another and to the writing of the other contributors. I was especially impressed with the creative ways that many of these women not only coped with challenging aspects of their personal life and work environments but found ways to creatively utilise them as ongoing solution development opportunities.

Early in my career, I had the good fortune to meet two of the original developers of the Solution Focused approach, Insoo Kim Berg and Eve Lipchik. Both remarkable women have had a significant influence on my way of working and teaching: Eve primarily through her scholarly writings and Insoo by virtue of spending many hours observing her work, doing Solution Focused trainings together, and eventually co-authoring a book. I was therefore not one bit surprised to read that many of the women in this book had been similarly inspired. Luckily for all of us, Eve is contributing her own foreword to this book. But sadly, my friend Insoo died in 2007. Therefore, I decided to share a personal memory of her that furthered my understanding and appreciation of the Solution Focused approach.

It was the late 1990s. Both Insoo and I were working very hard. In addition to doing Solution Focused training, we each saw clients, and wrote articles and books on the approach. Both of our husbands complained that we were always working! But although Insoo was 17 years older than me, she somehow always managed to do far more teaching and writing than I did! To this day, I have never met anyone who worked as tirelessly and with as much passion and enthusiasm as Insoo. She and I had an ongoing joke that she was the world champion of "joie de travail".

One fall, Insoo and I arranged to do some Solution Focused training together in South Korea. A shared room had been arranged for us in a local women's college dormitory. Although our accommodation was small and somewhat cramped, neither of us considered this to be a problem. In addition to being longtime colleagues, we had by then become very good friends, frequently staying in each other's homes. We had become so comfortable with one another that we occasionally cleaned each other's kitchens during our visits.

On that trip to South Korea our primary goal was to train the country's women's shelter workers. At that time, the women's shelters were an important new addition to the resources then available to homeless women and children in South Korea. Prior to the opening of these shelters, which allowed women to come with their children, domestic abuse victims were oftentimes forced to remain in abusive relationships simply because they had nowhere else to go. Insoo and I were both very impressed with the caring and dedication of the women colleagues we met on that trip and moved by the stories they told about the women and children they were helping.

After Insoo and I completed the first section of our SF training, we had a free day. Neither of us was the type to sit around drinking tea and resting, so we decided to set off on foot to look for a place where I could buy a string of nice pearls for my mother. Seoul is a very large city, so we did quite a bit of walking, looking into store after store, until we finally found one that Insoo deemed as the kind of place that catered to locals rather than tourists.

Once inside we walked over to the jewellery counter. Insoo explained to the salesman that we were looking for a nice string of pearls suitable for a mature woman. When he responded, Insoo noticed that he had a Japanese accent, and she immediately began conversing with him in his native language. (She was fluent in Japanese as well as Korean and English.)

The salesman pulled out tray after tray of pearls, then reached into a drawer under the counter and pulled out a little bag containing yet another set of pearls. He emptied the bag into his hand and displayed a string of randomly sized pearls of all different sizes, shades, and shapes. He explained that the non-uniformly sized pearls were intended to demonstrate the higher quality of the uniformly sized and shaped ones in the display trays.

I selected a classic string of uniformly sized pearls for my mother and paid for them. Meanwhile, Insoo, who rarely had any interest in shopping and almost never bought anything for herself, had uncharacteristically fallen completely in love with the string of non-uniform pearls. "These are the ones I want to buy," she told the astonished salesman. "I like them because each one is different from all the others." After a bit of convincing, the salesman finally agreed to sell Insoo the non-uniformly sized pearls; she left the shop wearing them around her neck. It occurred to me at the time that Insoo appreciated those non-uniformly sized pearls in much the same way that she valued the distinctive personal strengths, resources, and life experiences that contributed to our clients' uniquely effective, highly personalized solutions.

As I read the descriptions of how each of the women in this book chose to utilise the Solution Focused approach in her own way, I was strongly reminded of the beauty of Insoo's special string of pearls and how each one somehow seemed to shine more brightly because of the juxtaposition of their differences and connection to the others.

It is obvious that none of the women in this book have fallen into the trap of valuing their own expertise over that of their clients or claiming that their own way of using the Solution Focused approach is the one and only "right way". In every case, regardless of personal style, cultural differences, and individual preferences, they demonstrate the kind of respectful, generative collaborative spirit that is at the very heart of the very best use of the Solution Focused approach. This book gives me hope for the future of the Solution Focused approach. Bravo!

Yvonne Dolan
Santa Fe, New Mexico
September 2023

Foreword by Jane Lethem

In *Women's Perspectives on the Solution Focused Approach: International Applications and Interventions*, Anne-Marie Wulf and Jacqui von Cziffra-Bergs have put together a groundbreaking book, drawing on the experiences of Solution Focused practitioners across the globe. Their approach combines scholarship, focus, empathy, warmth, and humour.

They invited 17 Solution Focused practitioners to each contribute a chapter. The introductory chapter opens with an appreciative, welcoming, and jaunty introduction to each of the authors, the country, and the setting in which they work. The editors share with the reader their approach to helping each author to structure their contribution by giving each one eight deceptively simple questions and requests. These explore aspects of gender and their relationship to working in a Solution Focused way. Each chapter ends with a co-constructed reflection, in which Anne-Marie and Jacqui discuss in detail their reactions and reflections regarding each author's answers. Their exchange is non-critical, respectful, and in keeping with the emotion expressed by the author.

Solution Focused therapy developed in the late 1980s and began to spread from the United States of America to the United Kingdom and Europe. Initially, key texts and training came from male practitioners who were in leadership roles in their organisations. In the UK, Solution Focused ideas were taken up by male and female practitioners in both child and adult mental health. Clinicians who were enthusiastic faced challenges from senior colleagues who found the ideas unconventional and unsettling. Problem-focused approaches to mental health prevailed for many years.

As Solution Focused ideas gained more followers, some highly influential women practitioners and writers brought fresh perspectives to the approach and particularly inspired and encouraged other women. It is no surprise to note the number among the 17 authors of this book who named Insoo Kim Berg, Yvonne Dolan, or Eve Lipchik as having influenced them. They have been role models to many of us.

Contributors to the book who live and practise in other countries, outside the USA, UK, and Europe, have named other women who have influenced them in their own context. Solution Focused approaches continue to develop in new settings. Readers get a glimpse of their working lives, their challenges, and those of their clients. Some work in settings that are dangerous because of religious tensions, persecution of the LGBTQ community, misogyny, or violence. The book does not shy away from ongoing injustices and threats; the challenge of delivering Solution Focused therapy in such circumstances is hard to contemplate. The courage and ingenuity of those whose chapters illustrate work that is making a positive difference deserves respect. It would be good to know more about their "women of influence".

Jane Lethem, London, UK
September 2023

Introduction

Welcome, everyone, these are your editors speaking. Welcome to this Boeing 787 HopeCatcher, going around the world in less than 200 pages. We have just left Copenhagen Airport, Kastrup en route to OR Tambo International Airport in Johannesburg. As this is an impressive and diverse round trip visiting different countries, encountering a variety of contexts, and meeting incredible women using the Solution Focused approach, we advise you to fasten your Solution Focused seat belt, put the Strength-based seat in an upright position, and ensure that all loose problem-saturated objects are placed in the overhead locker. We would like to remind you of our instruction brochure in the pocket in front of you that embraces a statement made by Jane Lethem (1994, p. 33) nearly 30 years ago, when she said that "much can be learned from female Solution Focused Brief Therapy practitioners". So, sit back, relax, and get ready to embark on a journey where we meet 17 fantastic women who share how they apply the Solution Focused approach in different contexts. We have asked all 17 female Solution Focused practitioners to reflect on the same eight questions/instructions, each describing how they work and how their gender influences their practice.

1. *Reflect on how your gender influences your work–life and being a Solution Focused practitioner.*
2. *What is your good reason for staying a Solution Focused practitioner?*
3. *What would others notice you doing that would tell them that you work from a Solution Focused approach?*
4. *Share an exercise that might be useful to other women practitioners.*
5. *Share how you adapt the approach and make it your own. Give us five characteristics that are a part of your Solution Focused DNA.*
6. *Which female practitioner inspires you and in which way?*
7. *What soft small notion would you encourage other women practitioners to embrace?*
8. *My best hopes for other female Solution Focused voices.*

DOI: 10.4324/9781003430254-1

As we journey from the North to the South, West to East, we would like to wish you a pleasant, surprising, and informative journey ahead, as you hear unknown women working in fascinating areas making their voices known.

We start our journey in Copenhagen, Denmark, with co-editors Anne-Marie Wulf, who runs the Danish Solution Focused Institute, and Jacqui von Cziffra-Bergs, who runs the Solution Focused Institute of South Africa. They will discuss their ideas and insights on the basic assumptions of what it is to **be** Solution Focused, to **do** Solution Focused practice, and to **apply** Solution Focused interventions. The subsequent chapters are a journey around the world making unknown female voices known.

The first stop on our journey is Santiago, the capital of Chile. Santiago has around 6.2 million citizens and a mild Mediterranean climate. The country is squeezed between the Andes Mountains to the east and the Pacific Ocean to the west. In Chile lives Andrea Sandoval and María Amelia Barrera Morales, both psychologists and Solution Focused therapists who work mainly with trauma, domestic violence, and sexual abuse. María Amelia runs CentroSol, which trains psychologists across South America in Solution Focused therapy. Andrea is a therapist, stand-up comic, and laugh yoga therapist. She intuitively incorporates an element of humour into her work and creates a parallel experience with her clients. Chapter 2 is a tragicomedy about the use of humour and Solution Focused therapy in the face of trauma.

Reaching Chapter 3, we fly from South America to Mexico City, Mexico. The mountains that surround the city act like the rim of a bowl and contribute to serious air pollution problems. In this city with so much crime lives Sofie Geisler, a Danish anthropologist working for a senatorial candidate on his political campaign. Sofie has managed to develop a Solution Focused conflict management approach in the Mexican legal system that offers conflict resolution instead of going to court. Sofie has been living in Mexico City for decades, working in management, organisational development, and the legal system. Chapter 3 is about her work in the field between governance and politics.

Our journey then takes us further north to the United States of America and we land in Dallas, Texas. Here we meet Rebekka Ouer, who is a family therapist, specialising in work within the LGBTQ community. Rebekka's practice is a rainbow signalling safety in the queer community, giving people permission to be themselves. Rebekka works with couples, families, and individuals, and sees people not as problematic but rather as hopeful. She is determined to create safe spaces for the LGBTQ community, which she explores in Chapter 4.

Then it's a short flight from Dallas to Denver, the state capital of Colorado, where Teri Pichot is based. Teri is an experienced psychotherapist and has worked extensively with individuals, couples, and families in distress for over 30 years. She has designed and implemented innovative programmes that utilise Solution Focused Brief Therapy with animals, specifically dogs. Teri brings an experienced soft touch, a gentle touch, to the Solution Focused approach as she shares her work on animal-assisted therapy with us in Chapter 5.

Leaving an unusually hot Colorado, the HopeCatcher then flies north to Canada where we meet Alesya Courtnage, a psychotherapist doing her doctorate in social work. Alesya is passionate about increasing the accessibility of mental health services. She is a Solution Focused practitioner who is hooked on the approach and uses it exclusively. Waiting lists for care and mental health services in Canada were extremely long and the Canadian government mandated that all public agencies change their waiting lists and allow mental health walk-ins. It is here, in the short-term Brief Therapy space, that Alesya found her passion for Single Session Therapy. She now trains thousands of people on Solution Focused Single Session Therapy, which she shares with us in Chapter 6.

Dear fellow travellers, as we journey across the Atlantic, hearing these wonderful women describe their work, we, the editors, would like to serve you some light reflective refreshments. We hope to connect the common factors upon which these female practitioners rely, reflect on what this says about how women practise the Solution Focused approach, integrate, build, and construct new possibilities, and ultimately re-share our realisations with current and upcoming women in our field. Our editors' co-constructive reflections are discussed in a dialogue next to our photos, to indicate who is speaking. The aim of this book is to inspire female practitioners to make the approach their own and inspire women in general to trust how they use and apply the approach. So, please prepare yourself for landing as we reach Europe and the wonderful women who work there.

Landing in Germany, at Bremen's small airport, it's time to stretch our legs and visit Katrin Bergen. Katrin offers assistance to schools in implementing the Solution Focused method "Working on What Works" (WOWW), designed for classroom teachers. She is the co-founder of the global network "SF in Schools" and does a lot of classroom coaching, as well as individual coaching with children. As a woman she feels she does not want to be centre stage, but rather loves bringing parents, teachers, social workers, and children together to help create a future-forward moving notion, which she explores in Chapter 7.

After reboarding, we fly to the south of Spain and meet Marie-Carmen Neipp, a psychologist and university lecturer at the Miguel Hernández University, in Alicante. Marie-Carmen focuses on doing research on Solution Focused therapy and has published several articles. She is passionate about the field of health psychology and is interested in how Solution Focused language and questions contribute to the field of health and wellness, as she shares in Chapter 8.

Flying north-east, we land in Bern, the capital of Switzerland, where Ursula Buhlmann is a child and adolescent psychiatrist. Ursula has adapted the Solution Focused approach to suit her therapeutic work with children, teens, and families. Ursula integrates a holistic perspective into her work, as well as a lot of creativity. She is passionate about having fun when working and aims to have a joyful day in her workplace and drive home happy. In Chapter 9, Ursula shares how she uses this fun, playful approach with children and adolescents.

A short flight takes us from Bern to Croatia, where Dragana Knezić, a psychologist, lives in a small village near Zagreb. Dragana is originally from Serbia and works with traumatised people and torture victims. Dragana considers herself a therapist, psychologist, helper, and human rights activist who works with the forgotten. She has spent the past 20 years working with the underprivileged, poor children in care, families at risk, and refugees. Dragana finds the Solution Focused approach an inspirational gamechanger, especially when there are so few therapists supporting and serving thousands of refugees. In Chapter 10, Dragana shares how she uses the approach in a group setting to serve and support forgotten, unwanted people doing therapy in forests, at railway stations, and in refugee camps.

Then it's off to Russian Olga Zotova, sociologist, psychotherapist, and dancer who lives in Tel Aviv, Israel but works with clients throughout Europe. She integrates the Solution Focused approach with Body Work, Free Dance, and Embodiment therapy and is the founder of BabyContact. Olga began integrating her love of dance with the Solution Focused approach when she ran a mother and infant group and has since used the approach as a base for supportive community work, especially for women and children. Olga shares how she invites ideas from other approaches into her work and how she integrates embodiment with Solution Focused therapy in Chapter 11.

A message to everyone: we are about to serve breakfast before landing in Asia on this long journey of hope and connection. As we travel across the globe we uncover how our gender influences how we work, how we apply the Solution Focused approach differently, how the sociocultural context in which we work forms part of our Solution Focused application, and what common characteristics form part of our Solution Focused DNA. Just before we land we would like to remind you that hope sprouts when you find commonalities, when you see yourself in others, and when you know there are others like you. This book aims to co-construct a sense of belonging that strengthens our self-image and works against loneliness and isolation. By reading about other women in the field using the Solution Focused approach, we hope to give all women the courage to stand up for themselves, to have faith and belief in themselves, and to develop their own style, whatever that might be. Let's prepare the cabin crew for landing.

Taking off in Tel Aviv, Israel, we have a flight of approximately nine-and-half hours before landing in Beijing, China, where we meet the impressive Julia Li Hongyan. Julia is a Kids' Skills coach who lives in Finland but works with children and schools in China and is very passionate about kids, women, and education. Working in China, she noticed how children and parents were struggling and found her purpose in coaching parents, school teachers, and children. Julia shares her incredible work in Chapter 12.

A five-hour flight over the South China Sea takes us to Singapore to meet Jane Tuomola, a doctor of clinical psychology. Jane is originally from the United Kingdom but lives and works in Singapore and has written about Solution Focused practice in Asia. She has over 15 years of experience in adult mental health and specialises in individual psychological therapy, couples therapy, and coaching. Jane's big passion, however, is supervision, which she offers to healthcare professionals and which she discusses in Chapter 13.

After a long flight of nine hours and 6,293 kilometres, we land in Sydney, Australia, where we meet Jacqui van de Velde. Jacqui is a teacher and economist who works in well-being and, in particular, with veterans, veteran causes, and advocacy in the veteran space. Jacqui has found that the veteran support area is dominated by men, which presents challenges to women working in this field. Jacqui is passionate about using Solution Focused language in changing how people interact and have conversations to bring about change, especially in institutionalised areas such as the military. In Chapter 14 Jacqui shares her adventures in veteran support and how she applies the Solution Focused approach in a positive and life-giving way, creating disruptive thinking.

Yet another long flight takes us to the southernmost part of our journey as we land at Hawkés Bay Airport, New Zealand and meet Emma Burns, a psychologist and competitive swimmer. Emma works with the New Zealand Police and has developed a Solution Focused coaching framework for police officers to assist people affected by suicide. Emma offers Solution Focused suicide prevention workshops to both professionals and the general public and has most recently been elected as head of the Australian Solution Focused Association. Emma shares her insights and her voice with us on how to mainstream the Solution Focused approach in Chapter 15.

Can we have your attention, please, as we are now en route to our final round-trip destination – Johannesburg, South Africa. We want to thank you for flying with the HopeCatcher and becoming part of our Solution Focused family. Before you disembark, we would like to invite you to take all meaningful information with you.

Flying across the Indian Ocean to the southernmost part of Africa we meet Zibeth Hansen, a clinical psychologist with a degree in criminology who works for the Department of Correctional Services in a maximum-security prison outside Cape Town, South Africa. Zibeth is one of only two women at the prison, which houses only male offenders, and finds herself in a male-dominated environment. Zibeth uses the Solution Focused approach in her counselling with offenders in both individual sessions and group sessions and shares how she applies it in Chapter 16.

We have only two hours to fly up north to Johannesburg, where we meet Dr Zubeda Dragnor, a clinical psychologist who runs a women's shelter that protects and supports women who have experienced domestic violence. Zubeda uses a Solution Focused approach at the women's shelter and has trained all her staff in the Solution Focused approach, as she believes it creates hope and encourages the women to think of a different future. As a practising Muslim, Zubeda finds the Solution Focused approach very attractive as it aligns with her spiritual values. She shares her journey with us in Chapter 17.

Here we disembark and end our journey with a reflective summary in Chapter 18, written by our two editors, Jacqui and Anne-Marie. After hearing all the wonderful women's voices around the world, the editors have compiled a co-constructive reflection of learning and insight. The editors met at Mabula Game Lodge, north of Johannesburg, ending and concluding this book by asking themselves: What are the commonalities? What are the golden threads? What has surprised us? What has stood out for us on this journey? What does our Solution Focused DNA look like and how do we apply it?

We are incredibly proud to be part of this fabulous Solution Focused family and our hope is that you join us. We feel humble and grateful to belong to such a wonderful, empowered community. In describing our unique Solution Focused DNA, our best hope is that this helps you reflect on your **being** and **doing** in order to discover your own unique Solution Focused DNA.

Our best hope is, as you journey with us and meet these fabulous women, that you not only learn from them but also find their voices as a guiding light. We hope this book helps you, the reader, become a supporter, a surpriser, a safe haven, an advocate, a server and helper, an awareness giver, and a gamechanger.

Disclaimer: this book is not only for female readers and practitioners. Everybody can be inspired by reading about how the Solution Focused practice unfolds in so many different contexts.

Reference

Lethem, J. (1994). *Moved to tears, moved to action: Solution Focused Brief Therapy with women and children.* BT Press.

Chapter 1

Our Solution Focused DNA

How the being, the doing, and the context influence our implementation and application

Anne-Marie Wulf (Denmark) and
Jacqui von Cziffra-Bergs (South Africa)

Copenhagen
Wednesday, 2 March 2022

Dear Jacqui
I'm not sure we have met yet; however, I'm aware of your huge work in South Africa and that you're an experienced SF practitioner in terms of working with traumatised people. The European Brief Therapy Association (EBTA), of which I'm a board member, has received a request from the Russian SF Association. The request has been handed over to me as head of the International Cooperation Task Group (ICTG) under EBTA. We have decided to contact experienced practitioners with the necessary knowledge that's requested. Our Russian friends ask if anyone is willing to do some training, a workshop, for free. They need knowledge, ideas, tips, and tricks (my words) to manage the situation they're in, seeing traumatised families, clients, and victims.

If you're willing to do something, I'll pass on your email to our colleagues and they will contact you and coordinate.

Looking forward to hearing from you.
Warmly,
Anne-Marie

Johannesburg
Thursday, 3 March 2022

Dear Anne-Marie
So good to make contact with you (albeit under such sad conditions). I will gladly help and share with the SF community in Russia and Europe. They are very welcome to contact me and I will see if I can assist in any way. Would love to meet up with you in person or we can at some point set up a Zoom meet-and-greet coffee chat.

Talk to you soon,
Jacqui

DOI: 10.4324/9781003430254-2

Finding a friend

Paradoxically, a conflict in one part of the world resulted in two women from totally different parts of the world, Denmark and South Africa, connecting and finding incredible common ground, not only in wanting to help others but also in our love for the Solution Focused approach. An email from the North (the Danish Solution Focused Institute) was answered by an email from the South (the Solution Focused Institute of South Africa). A distance of 13,477 km separated us and yet there was an instant connection, instant recognition, and a mutual understanding embedded in the Solution Focused approach. Within less than 24 hours we had established a relationship, not really knowing the impact we would have on each other's lives.

Meeting regularly over Zoom, we drank a lot of coffee and tea, had moments of fun, laughter, and joy, and discovered a mutual passion for and fascination with the Solution Focused approach and life in general. Our conversations were naturally and instinctively built upon the basic assumptions and values of the Solution Focused approach, as we both constantly acknowledged each other's situations, showed immense respect, unconditionally trusted each other, and built our conversations on kind-humility. This made it easy to create interesting dialogues, not only about the Solution Focused approach but also about what we had in common, seeing glimpses of ourselves in the other as daughters of elderly mothers with special-care needs that we, as daughters, were expected to meet. Female perspectives were shared, and an idea arose. What if we could put together a book in which more female perspectives and voices from other female Solution Focused practitioners could be heard? Steve de Shazer (1988, p. 6) writes about the solution always standing in the shadow of the problem, the hidden other, and this made us think about how female Solution Focused practitioners have been standing in the shadows, quietly going about their work and yet not given an opportunity to be heard. We became curious about the possibility of women sharing their ideas and experiences and we became excited about discovering unknown Solution Focused female voices, hearing their descriptions of where they work and especially how they are utilising the Solution Focused approach in their own unique ways.

As we took the very first and smallest steps toward the idea of writing a book proposal, we began recording our Zoom meetings, and have done so continuously since the autumn of 2022, over time adding drawings on the Zoom whiteboard to express ourselves, explain and demonstrate our ideas, and start reflecting on the creation of new ideas. What transpired between us during this year is a true reflection of what the Solution Focused approach is all about: two people listening with intentional caring and interest, asking each other beautiful questions, building and creating useful ideas together, constantly co-constructing new understandings, and doing it with true caring in a playful, fun way. Each Zoom meeting was so indicative of what the Solution Focused approach is all about that both of us realised that something incredible was happening. We realised that our connection was based on the same embedded assumptions and theory of Solution Focused thinking, and that we were connecting from the same platform.

Our connection was firmly built on two things – first, we are both women; and second, we are both Solution Focused thinkers and practitioners. Yes, we all know that Solution Focused practice is an approach to helping people, yet every person who becomes Solution Focused very quickly realises that it becomes a life philosophy (Kim et al., 2017; Burgstaller et al., 2019; Burns, 2021). This embedded similarity, our gender and our approach, made us curious and excited and led to many questions: What role does gender play in how we work? How would other women describe their experiences of being women in the Solution Focused field? What are our common assumptions about the Solution Focused approach? How do we as women practise using the Solution Focused approach?

Our assumptions

Our experiences, discoveries, and reflections on the life we have lived influence the way we act and behave. We live life, and with it we constantly gain new experience, and therefore continuously revise and construct assumptions about situations and other people. We talk about life being a social construct where we develop and change through relationships, experiences, and reflections (Gergen, 1997). If we believe and trust that a small child can ride a bicycle by herself, then we act in a way that encourages a positive outcome. This means that we do not interfere or put our hand on her back; rather we behave in a way that ensures that she succeeds. Instead of interfering or holding her for support, or controlling the situation, we trust the child to do it by herself. Our inner life has an outer expression, and vice versa. Our values and beliefs will influence how we interact and behave in the world and ultimately shape reality (Brelnes, 2015). Burgstaller et al. (2019) describe the Solution Focused approach as consisting of the *beings* (the beliefs and values) and the *doings* (how we act and what we do). To this we add a third component – *time*, which is the journey and context that contributes to who we are and serves as a dynamic co-creative factor. As Solution Focused practitioners our beliefs (*being*) are the same, embedded and rooted in Solution Focused principles. Our *doing* is based on what we believe and influences our actions; thus the way we *do* Solution Focused is unique. Our *time*, our context and journey, is uniquely our own, shaped by the way we have lived and our lives, and is formed by our experiences and relationships, thus who we have become and who we are.

So, what does **being** Solution Focused mean and what lies at the core of our **being** Solution Focused? As trainers and practitioners, we would be pleased if our participants and clients noticed the following:

- A shift in perspective from a problem orientation towards a solution focus. It is all about "Solution building" (Kim et al., 2017, p. 17) rather than problem solving; about exploring current resources and future hopes instead of the causes of the problem (Bannink, 2014). As Denise Yusuf says, it is a shift from the "why" of failure to the "how to" of success (2021, p. 2); it is a "welcome alternative" (Kim et al., 2017, p. 28).

- All people have ideas about what they want and what is good for them, and we are all motivated for something, and thus each person is the expert of her own life (Metcalf, 2008; Fiske, 2018; Conniff, 2021; Metcalf, 2021).
- All people have resources, competence, and skills; however, they might not know or see it for themselves yet. Solution Focused practitioners see clients as capable and as having all the resources and abilities within themselves to change (Bannink, 2014). All clients have "unique and individual talents and strengths" (Watson & Birkett, 2021, p. 88).
- Change is always happening (Fiske, 2018); it is constant and inevitable. As Solution Focused practitioners our role is to enhance the fact that things are already changing and focus on one small step that leads to bigger steps of change (Lipchik, 2011; King, 2017), taking "small steps forward to the joy of life" (Dierolf, 2014, p. 33).

Our **doings** are led by the **beings**, and cause us to:

- Create a collaborative and co-constructive dialogue with our clients where we "co-construct new meaning" (Franklin, 2018), helping our clients see themselves and their lives differently. For us Solution Focused practice is an approach with a set stance toward our client and how we cooperate with our client (Lipchik, 2009), constantly co-constructing the conversation (King, 2021a) and focusing on what people are doing to get through difficult situations (Conniff, 2021) in order to build on "descriptions of preferred future experiences" (Barnai & Soregi, 2021, p. 133).
- Ask questions rather than give advice, and thus use questions that allow the client to reflect and find their inner wisdom. As Fredrike Bannink states, "[W]e live in worlds our questions create" (2014, p. 52) and as Solution Focused practitioners we ask questions that steer the conversation into actively shaping a new version of the client's life. Our questions "are effective in bringing ideas to life" (Conniff, 2021, p. 114).
- Pay attention and listen constructively (Fiske, 2018) for the client's strengths, capacities, and good reasons; hear what is working and what the client wants in the future. This is a conversation with a constant pivot between acknowledging the difficulty and validating strengths and resilience (King, 2021b). As Solution Focused practitioners we all listen constructively, we select in our own individual and unique ways, and we build based on our selection (Lipchik, 2011; King, 2017).
- Use hope-catching language that is a light "tap on the shoulder" toward hope and change (Fiske, 2018, p. 66). We are mindful of our language and how we use language to create a different linguistic reality for the client (de Shazer & Dolan, 2007) where "tomorrow turns out to be a better day" (Conniff, 2021, p. 111) and creates a "hopeful, almost expectant tone" (Kim et al., 2017, p. 19).

Our Solution Focused DNA

Our embedded assumptions inform how we practise the Solution Focused approach. Four *beings* that inform four *doings* done in our own unique **time and context** result in our own unique Solution Focused DNA. Our personalities, our experiences, and our relationships all inform our *being* and *doing* and build our unique Solution Focused DNA. A walk down memory lane reminds us of the people we have met along the way, the impact they have had, the training and workshops we have attended and participated in, the words we have written, the language we have spoken; all contributing to our unique ways of applying the Solution Focused approach, our own contextual Solution Focused DNA, and our good reasons for staying Solution Focused.

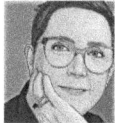 For me, Anne-Marie, my grandfather had a significant impact on my life. He worked with children in foster care and his actions and behaviour showed me the basic values of solidarity, caring for people in need, respect, and the right to express oneself. It was quite late in life that I realised the huge impact he had on me and how these values have become my guiding star, and in many ways fit so well with the basic Solution Focused assumptions. During my Solution Focused journey since 2003, I have been walking the path of training with my soulmate Karin Pharés, with whom I studied the diploma programme at SIKT in Malmö. These trips to Malmö contributed decisively to reflection on and development and implementation of the Solution Focused approach through a co-constructive and collaborative process. Our reflections and talks are still so valuable to me as we continue this journey by attending conferences and workshops, or just sharing a cup of coffee.

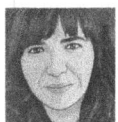 And for me, Jacqui, my South African heritage and context inform how I think about and approach life. Growing up in South Africa has undoubtedly influenced how I do life. Being honest, practical, and having a fundamental mindset of "if something is not working you make a plan" are the foundation that resonates with *being* Solution Focused. Living in an area where problems are abundant and yet constantly bearing witness to the resilience of people, the creativity of people, and the hopefulness that people have has formed part of my DNA. I have also been fortunate to meet and work with another Solution searcher in the form of my friend Merritt Watson. Merritt's constant reminders of "How are we going to do differently here?" and "Where are the wows in this situation?" have definitely contributed to my Solution Focused mindset.

MY SOLUTION FOCUSED DNA: A TRIP DOWN MEMORY LANE

Imagine walking down memory lane as you pass people who have influenced your life, your beliefs, your behaviour.

You pass the bookshop, you stop and look in the window at the books, all from your life, professional and private, schools and education.

You slowly move on and discover a man miming some of the situations you've been in, parodying former colleagues in a gentle and soft way.

You buy an ice cream, and as you watch the mime, you reflect on your SF DNA - what has contributed to "Present Moments", the journey you've been on so far? What books or articles have had a significant impact? Who has inspired you most and in what way? What would your three simple Beings and Doings sound like?

Looking at our practice, we will without a doubt discover that even though our mutual Solution Focused *being* is the same, our Solution Focused *doing* has commonalities *but* differs slightly, based on our *time and context*. Our different contexts and life experiences will surely influence how we ask questions, how we respond, and how we formulate language (De Jong et al., 2013), and perhaps our gender, the fact that we are all women, also shapes and influences the way in which we use and apply the Solution Focused approach. So, on reflection, how does our gender influence our work life and being Solution Focused?

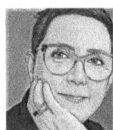

It's definitely a difficult question to answer. I have given it a lot of consideration and still am, I guess. It would have been easier to ask my clients how they feel, think about, and observe my gender influencing my work and collaboration with them. They might say something about a gentle, caring attitude, where I lean forward, waiting and yet curiously inviting them to share. Patiently waiting with long pauses for the smallest sign of response, not afraid of or avoiding emotions, accepting that I get emotional too. I imagine having a strong intuition helping and telling me how to act and what to do in my practice as well in my private life, which often allows me to improvise. And maybe, reflecting on this question, my gender also has an impact on my outer attitude, the way I stand in larger groups, or the way I dress or act as a woman. It reminds me of hearing Insoo Kim Berg once saying, regarding the distinction between coaching and therapy: in coaching you put on a business suit – and in some contexts I consciously put on a business suit, e.g. negotiating a contract. Being a Solution Focused practitioner, the beliefs and assumptions "run in my veins" and have had an impact on my personal relationships and my motherhood. I recall my youngest daughter at age 12 arguing with her father and suddenly saying: "So, what difference would it make if I put on a jacket?", and I smiled in the back, because strong communication skills are an important and great side effect of the Solution Focused approach.

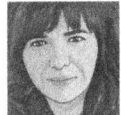

For me, Jacqui, being a woman definitely influences how I work. I feel that I can sit with heavy and hard emotions for a long time, because emotions do not scare me. I see being emotional and being vulnerable as part of a healing process. Also, as a mother I am continuously making it up as I go along. Motherhood did not come with a manual, so there are often times I just go with my gut and do and say what feels best in the moment. I do the same as a practitioner; I just intuitively go with what my gut tells me to do. I was made an associate professor at a very early age and there was an old established male professor who made my life hell. He used to make a point of calling me "girlie" in front of colleagues or saying things like "Women will never understand what it means to be serious". Without realising it he played a major role in me becoming a little rebellious and silently defiant, nearly helping to create a mindset of "I will show you, I can". This quiet rebellion to not accept the negative is something I hold on to as a therapist. I suppose I quietly rebel against accepting that my clients are victims and keep searching for the survivor in them. This helps me stay a strength searcher, a resilience seeker, and a possibility facilitator.

Summary

Indistinguishably our gender influences our lives and our work, and, maybe not surprisingly, we both mention how being mothers contributes to our Solution Focused DNA and how we both use a small soft touch called our intuition. This leads us to encourage other female Solution Focused practitioners to embrace their gut feelings. Your intuition is like an internal GPS, with your instincts giving signs or hints about everything, such as the decisions you make, ways to act, or actions to take. Everyone has natural instincts that are present – this is not intrinsically linked to having children; rather it is about listening to your inner voice. This book is about women sharing their voice in a context of working as Solution Focused practitioners, yet all of us also have our own internal voice, guiding us in life and work. As Denise Yusuf (2021, p. 6) says so beautifully, "waiting for certainty" is a waste, and as practitioners we go on a journey of co-creating with our clients, doing what works in the moment and trying new things out (Burns, 2021).

London
Friday, 17 February 2023

Dear Jacqui and Anne-Marie
It gives me great pleasure to inform you that the members of our Editorial Board unanimously and enthusiastically approved your project this morning.
Many congratulations! I am confident your new book will make a terrific addition to Routledge's publishing programme, and I am thrilled to be working with you.

Best,
Grace McDonnell
Routledge

References

Bannink, F. (2014). *Post traumatic success*. W.W. Norton & Company.
Barnai, A., & Soregi, V. (2021). Facing new challenges using the Solution Focused approach. In D. Yusuf (Ed.), *The Solution Focused approach with children and young people*. Routledge.
Brelnes, J. (2015, 30 August). Three ways your beliefs can shape your reality. *Psychology Today*. https://www.psychologytoday.com/za/blog/in-love-and-war/201508/3-ways-your-beliefs-can-shape-your-reality
Burns, E. (2021). Using the Solution Focused approach within the New Zealand Police to create happy endings for young people. In D. Yusuf (Ed.), *The Solution Focused approach with children and young people*. Routledge.
Burgstaller, S., Iveson, I., & Karrer, H. (2019). *Team talk: Building excellence with Solution Focused skills*. www.teamtalk.usolvit.com
Conniff, H. (2021). Solution Focused injections. In D. Yusuf (Ed.), *The Solution Focused approach with children and young people* (pp. 108–115). Routledge.
De Jong, P., Bavelas, J.B., & Kormann, H. (2013). An introduction to using microanalysis to observe co-construction in psychotherapy. *Journal of Systemic Therapies, 32*(3), s. 17–30.
De Shazer, S. (1988). *Clues: Investigating solutions in Brief Therapy*. W.W. Norton & Company.
De Shazer, S., & Dolan, Y. (2007). *More than miracles*. Routledge.
Dierolf, K. (2014). *Solution Focused team coaching*. SolutionsAcademy.
Fiske, H. (2018). Preventing trauma in the aftermath of trauma. In A. Froerer (Ed.), *SFBT and clients managing trauma.* (pp. 64–84). Oxford University Press.
Franklin, C. (2018). *Solution Focused Brief Therapy in alternative schools*. Routledge.
Gergen, K. (1997). *Realities and relationships: Soundings in social construction*. Harvard University Press.

Kim, J., Kelly, M., & Franklin, C. (2017). *Solution Focused Brief Therapy in schools*. Oxford University Press.

King, P. (2017). *Tools for effective therapy with children and families*. Routledge.

King, P. (2021a). Solution Focused play therapy. In D. Yusuf (Ed.), *The Solution Focused approach with children and young people* (pp. 15–21). Routledge.

King, P. (2021b). Yes … and … In D. Yusuf (Ed.), *The Solution Focused approach with children and young people* (pp. 156–161). Routledge.

Lipchik, E. (2009). A Solution Focused journey. In E. Connie (Ed.), *The art of Solution Focused therapy* (pp. 45–64). Springer Publishing.

Lipchik, E. (2011). *Beyond technique in Solution-Focused therapy: Working with emotions and the therapeutic relationship*. The Guilford Press.

Metcalf, L. (2021). A Solution Focused team conversation. In D. Yusuf (Ed.), *The Solution Focused approach with children and young people* (pp. 72–78). Routledge.

Metcalf, M. (2008). *Counselling toward solutions*. Jossey-Bass.

Watson, M., & Birkett, N. (2021). Dream … believe … achieve. In D. Yusuf (Ed.), *The Solution Focused approach with children and young people* (pp. 87–94). Routledge.

Yusuf, D. (Ed.) (2021). *The Solution Focused approach with children and young people*. Routledge.

Chapter 2

Addressing trauma through Solution Focused Brief Therapy in Chile

Two female voices from the South

María Amelia Barrera Morales and
Andrea Sandoval Riquelme (Chile)

Introduction

In 2015, María Amelia Barrera Morales founded Centro Sol, the Institute of Solution Focused Brief Therapy in Latin America. María Amelia wanted to create an organisation that teaches and trains therapists in Spanish, and to establish a place of learning and sharing. Owing to the harsh and often traumatic context in which Chilean clients find themselves, María Amelia decided that Solution Focused Brief Therapy was a good fit and another way to understand and work with people managing trauma. Andrea Sandoval Riquelme joined as a co-presenter in 2020 and together they not only offer Solution Focused training courses for psychologists, schools, protection centres, and municipalities, but also conduct research.

Reflect on how your gender influences your work–life and being a Solution Focused practitioner

A survey done by the Department of Health (Superintendencia de Salud, 2022) in Chile indicated that, of 72,795 registered psychologists, 73% were women and only 27% men. In Latin America, as in the rest of the world, biological sex and its respective roles have been associated with behavioural characteristics that are often rooted in culture. Our culture usually assigns the responsibility of care and the treatment of emotional issues, which tend to be viewed as private, to the feminine role. This results in the development of certain characteristics such as empathy, active listening, receptivity, the ability to understand and communicate emotions, emotional containment, and an eagerness to help. These characteristics correspond to those required by a psychologist, especially for one working in a clinical field, and it is thus a great advantage that most psychologists are female.

María Amelia

The different demands on women to balance family life and work life and make these compatible have led me to choose to teach and stay in private practice. This prompted me to start Centro Sol, an organisation that teaches and trains

DOI: 10.4324/9781003430254-3

psychologists in Solution Focused Brief Therapy. Cento Sol has nurtured and facilitated my professional growth and, at the same time, has trained and developed a different generation of psychologists. Centro Sol has become a place for therapists to meet and collaborate; it is also a well-walked and worthy path for me that has incorporated new female voices into the Solution Focused approach.

Andrea

My sensitivity to gender inequality and male dominance in the development of psychological theory has resulted in a personal rebellion and a desire for female voices and perspectives to be made known and take a place of relevance. The place of women in psychology can no longer be that of being seen as "hysterical" case studies who fantasise about their own abuse.

As two female therapists working in Chile, the context of our country and the cultural view of women have influenced us both. Chile has a history of harsh, traumatic situations: a 17-year dictatorship, a rugged geography prone to natural disasters, social inequality, conflicts over ownership of land claimed by native ethnic groups, rising immigration, and high rates of violence against women and children. All of this makes working with trauma unavoidable and an imperative focus. For us, Solution Focused Brief Therapy is simultaneously an efficient and empathic perspective; it is respectful and validating, it is delicate and connected with hope, and it works with people who have suffered trauma. As therapists working mainly with trauma, this is a good reason for us to have chosen the Solution Focused approach above any other.

What is your good reason for staying a Solution Focused practitioner?

- It truly works in a short period of time. Several authors, among them Neipp and Beyebach (2022), conclude that this model has proven to be effective, is cross-culturally adaptive, and effective regardless of the format in which it is applied.
- It's a kind approach; respectful, positive, and hopeful.
- It's an ethical model: it reduces the possibility of re-victimisation by not focusing on the problem and trauma; and it diminishes suffering by putting clients in charge of their change and their recovery.
- Clients learn to take care of themselves, they are empowered without having to rely on the therapist, and they are able to develop a more compassionate and validating posture.
- It allows the therapist to be affected positively and develop vicarious resilience (Froerer et al., 2018).

These good reasons not only led us to choose Solution Focused Brief Therapy but also makes us marvel at how compatible it is in trauma-related situations.

What would others notice you doing that would tell them that you work from a Solution Focused approach?

What students and clients are already noticing and commenting on is the active listening, the validation, the hopeful environment we set, the permanent focus on the positive, and the variety of questions about the future. People will also notice that we have a resource focus and that we recognise what clients do well. We have genuine confidence in our clients' capabilities and potential. This allows the clients to see their issues from a different viewpoint and to leave the first session already slightly relieved and with significant ideas for change.

Share an exercise that might be useful to other women practitioners

Green flags and red flags

In working with people who have suffered traumatic situations and are still at risk, the concept of "safety signals" is fundamental. According to Pérez (2006, p. 50), trauma "breaks one or more of the basic assumptions that constitute the safety references of the human being, and especially the beliefs of invulnerability and control over life itself". That is why it is important to help clients who have suffered traumatic experiences to progressively recover the ability to be an agent for their own safety. Dolan (1991) and Turnell and Edwards (1999) agree on the necessity of working with techniques such as safety scaling and safety signals, establishing safety goals, measuring the current safety levels of the client and their family, and determining what are the best indicators of safety. The commonly used concepts of "red flags" and "green flags" are given to survivors of trauma in order to perform this exercise.

First, when talking about the issue, the information given by the client is spontaneously organised under the concept of "red flags", and the new safety signals, which we co-construct, under the concept of "green flags". We start by saying something like, "I've listened to you carefully, and from what you have told me, there's a lot of clarity about the danger signals, the 'red flags', if you're okay with calling them that [wait for the client's approval before using this concept]. You have also learned how to detect them, and what to do when they appear, which is good! What signs or 'green flags' will allow you to realise that you are safe and sound?"

Given that, in general, the client will not have thought of this, it can be a difficult question to answer. Often, looking for opposites to or antonyms of their "red flags" helps them elaborate on their answers. It is important to dig deeper and make it personal by unpacking the opposites with specific significance and "difference" questions. A visual reminder can be useful, for example sticking a red flag on one wall and a green flag on another, writing down a list underneath each one, and then inviting the client to recognise some of the safety indicators that might be present in their lives.

Share how you adapt the approach and make it your own. Give us five characteristics that are a part of your Solution Focused DNA

María Amelia

For people going through traumatic situations, the traditional model taught by De Jong and Berg (2013) works best for me. The most important thing is to build trust, which in the context of trauma is often slow. The phrase "the person is the centre of everything, not the trauma" is always a guiding force for me. I actively listen for signs of light from the client and begin with the question, "What would need to happen here so that, when you leave, you can say it was worth your time, that the time you spent here has been worthwhile for you?" (De Shazer et al., 2007). This is a respectful invitation of hope. Part of my DNA is selectively and explicitly high-lighting resources and ways of coping, showing surprise at this coping and trying to, if possible, get a smile from the client. In trauma work, "the desired future" is done as an in-session activity. Saying, for example, "It's difficult, the things you've gone through, and it shows your [inserting and utilising the client's language]. It's very important that you have a clear written log of how you are feeling and what you will be doing differently, when you feel free of those tormenting memories." I believe that understanding that the traumatic event has occurred, that it is not going to go away, is important. However, we can help clients do things differently, for example by asking, "What would tell you that you are ready to work on it? What would tell you that you are dealing better with it?" Highlighting conversations about exceptions when the desired future has already been described is very helpful and I finish every session by talking about what we have taken from the conversation that has been useful. This allows the client to organise the things we have talked about.

Andrea

The first component of my Solution Focused DNA is that I tune in to my setting and adjust how I show respect to the client by allowing them to preserve their dignity. Secondly, I take it easy in the sessions and go slowly. These personal manoeuvres correspond with the posture of the Solution Focused therapist, and they contribute to what Lipchick (2004) calls the *emotional climate* necessary for therapy to develop properly. The third component of my Solution Focused DNA is that I create opportunities for resources and solutions to emerge and I take advantage of these resources to enable the client to connect with possible solutions. Having this as my North, I improvise and use any technique to build and connect the client to their resources. I believe that the more emphasis is placed on this, the more the client will feel a sense of capability and agency, and the faster the therapy process will be. Finally, to normalise I use humour whenever possible. Various authors point out that the use of humour in working with trauma is helpful (Fry & Salameh, 2004; Pérez, 2006; Vanistendael et al., 2013; Furman, 2013,

2018). Humour is the shining light and illuminates resilience and coping. Given the spontaneous emergence of humour in interactions with clients, it is difficult to describe the structure and guiding principles of using humour. However, respect for the client's personality, style, and pace is helpful. I often follow this sequence in a session: normalisation, recovery scale, and resource talk. This allows the client to reframe their understanding, frees them from the strong problem focus, and allows them to evaluate their progress more positively, while recognising the resources they have already used.

Which female practitioner inspires you and in which way?

María Amelia

Learning with Teri Pichot and being charmed by her style is easy. While taking classes with her, I came to understand the essence of Solution Focused Brief Therapy. I admire the depth of her knowledge, the clarity of the model's essence, her shining a light on the truly important parts, her smooth style, her respect, her subtlety, and her precision. The way in which she develops Solution Focused Brief Therapy with people at social risk (Pichot & Dolan, 2003) and in cases of addiction (Pichot & Smock, 2009) – maintaining respect towards the clients and avoiding judgement, always seeing the best in them – has had a profound impact on me.

Andrea

Yvonne Dolan is one of the main developers of the Solution Focused approach and she inspires me immensely. She has walked a long road in working with a difficult client population. Her work with victims of sexual abuse has made it clear that Solution Focused Brief Therapy is effective in complex cases. She has also developed intervention strategies that are useful in applying the Solution Focused approach to all kinds of traumatic experiences. She has been my inspiration since 2004, when I first specialised in sexual abuse and began reading her work. It was my first contact with Solution Focused Brief Therapy and I am eternally grateful for it.

What soft small notion would you encourage other women practitioners to embrace?

We would like to encourage other female practitioners to recognise everything they are doing right and that works. Recognise what is working and do more of it. Also, if a resource emerges, use it. Utilising resources is powerful, so do it, and you will see how things change.

My best hopes for other female Solution Focused voices

Nuestra mejor esperanza para las voces de otras practicantes centradas en soluciones es que:

- Las voces crezcan y se multipliquen
- Sus voces también sean escuchadas
- Ellas oigan su propia voz con respeto, amor, aceptación incondicional, con tanto compromiso con ellas mismas como lo tienen por otros
- Se validen a sí mismas, sean claras y firmes aún ante el embate de voces que se arroguen el protagonismo y la apropiación de lo cierto
- Que estas voces se asocien con otras voces femeninas compartiendo saberes, generando nuevas comprensiones y aplicaciones para el enfoque centrado en soluciones
- Con respeto y valoración a la diversidad, elaborando e integrando los aportes, generando una armonía coral

Our best hopes for the voices of other Solution Focused practitioners are that:

- Their voices grow and multiply;
- Their voices are heard and made known;
- They hear their own voices with the same respect, love, unconditional acceptance, and commitment to themselves that they have for others;
- They validate themselves by remaining firm and clear even before an onslaught of voices that contradict them or steal their true selves;
- Their voices are associated with other female voices sharing knowledge and generating new understanding and new applications of the Solution Focused model; and
- They respect and validate diversity, and elaborate on and integrate all contributions into a harmonious chorus.

Co-constructive editors' reflection

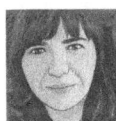

These two women have done something remarkable – they have created a Solution Focused organisation in a part of South America that is riddled with trauma. All by themselves, with limited resources and allies, they've established a community of Solution Focused thinkers to support and guide clients through trauma. They really have done a lot with a little, doing this on their own and creating a meeting place for like-minded therapists to empower clients.

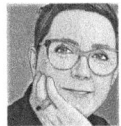

Yes, looking at the journey these two women have taken in this harsh and traumatic context, and doing it on their own, is remarkable, Jacqui, a little bit like you have done too, because there is a huge difference between someone in Europe who has all the resources and a supportive community and someone in South America or South Africa who has no one to turn to and are on their own.

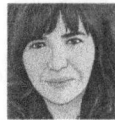

And then there were the descriptions of how culture plays a significant role in the roles we play as women and how these roles seem to align with the qualities needed to be a therapist. I also appreciated the comments about how motherhood and running a family has a significant impact on our career choices and how we are constantly trying to balance family and work life. I also love that they chose Solution Focused Brief Therapy very intentionally as their therapeutic approach in working with trauma: as they say so beautifully, it is delicate and empathic.

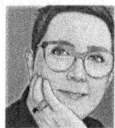

Yes, they have intentionally chosen Solution Focused therapy to use in their context, as it makes more sense than other approaches.

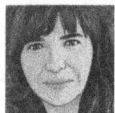

Yes, as all their cases present with some form of trauma and they find the Solution Focused approach respectful and hopeful. When you work with trauma, the element of hope is crucial and the Solution Focused approach is hope-giving. This chapter made me think that our work with trauma is not about trauma debriefing but rather about a "resilience rebrief" (Froerer et al., 2018, p. 49). Debriefing trauma builds a relationship with the trauma and we want to build a relationship with a resilient version of the client. I love that for these two ladies the emphasis is on putting their clients back in charge of change and recovery.

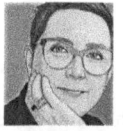

I really like that they have this emphasis on empowering the client, and as therapists they take this very special stance, this stance of empowering the client rather than taking over the trauma or even taking over the healing.

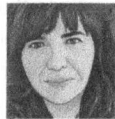

Yes, we have to remember they are listening to trauma on a daily basis and that working in a hope-giving Solution Focused way is good for the clients and good for the therapist, preventing therapist burnout (Froerer et al., 2018). They constantly have a resource focus and look for change and recovery. I love that they enter trauma with a resource focus because it empowers the client and saves the therapist. I love their permanent focus on the positive and on questions that link to the future. The golden nugget of this chapter is asking clients what they did well because clients managing trauma do not feel they do anything well, clients who are battered by trauma forget they have done well. I love that they have a genuine confidence and fundamental belief in their clients as resourceful and capable.

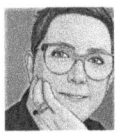

And I really like the idea of already in the first session focusing on strengthening, so the client leaves relieved and hopeful. Empowerment from the beginning. You get the impression that from the first minute of the first session they are focused on strengthening the client, and that is a really good idea.

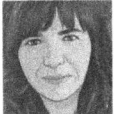

I love that the red and green flag exercise acknowledges what happened to the client and that we cannot change what happened, *but* we can change how we react to the triggers and memories. They are using flashbacks and red flags as safety signals. They are saying safety first and safety is possible, and safety is a process; thus recovery also happens on that continuum. I also love that they use the concept of asking the clients for opposites. When the client is stuck or overwhelmed by the trauma and cannot answer what they want instead, they ask the client what the opposite is of what they are feeling or experiencing. This is very helpful, especially if the client is stuck in a trauma rut, and allows creative thinking to take place. I also love that the guiding force is the client and not the trauma story – very mindfully she searches for the person and not the trauma.

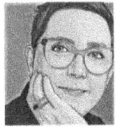

I really like the respectful invitation of hope – this is an invitation to look at trauma differently and is done in the direction of hope. This is their DNA and describes how they work. And I really love their concrete examples from practice, and got this feeling of being in the session with them. And then the metaphor of a compass impressed me: our true North is hope and the client's resources set the direction of the conversations. I like that if we stick to the course to the North, if we stick to this attitude, then the client's sense of capacity and capability increases, and the faster the process will be. And then I love how they say humour is the shining light. So I get this picture of my North, and the shining light of humour highlights it.

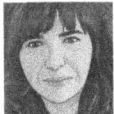

I get the feeling that part of their DNA is to tune in to the client and to dance and move with the client to preserve their dignity. She manoeuvres or dances in the emotional trauma climate, constantly containing the client's dignity but at the same time steering the dance toward resources and solutions. I also love that humour illuminates the resources and how she uses the bizarre, the ironic, as a tragic comedy and as a spontaneous resource. I love how they are constantly searching for the light in other female practitioners who write about the Solution Focused approach, how they search for light in their clients, how they are a light for each other and then also for us.

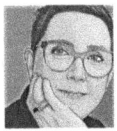

They are inviting us to notice what we are already doing right and to use resources to create powerful shifts. I love that their work is so inclusive of all cultures and creates a chorus of harmony.

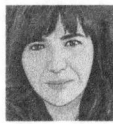 These two women have created a whole choir of Solution Focused practitioners where therapists can meet and share and learn from each other, and they are sharing and multiplying. They are inviting us to listen to each other and integrate our knowledge into a helpful song for others.

Author references

Barrera, M.A. (2018). Lo único constante es el cambio. Aprendizaje del modelo Centrado en Soluciones en un grupo de terapeutas. In F. García, C. Hernández, P. Arroyo & R. Mardones (Eds.), *Historias de cambio. El enfoque sistémico en acción* (pp. 387–389). UST/RIL editores.

Barrera, M.A., González, K., Carrasco, S., & Hernández, A. (2021, September-December). Pilot implementation of WOWW Program in a Chilean private school. *Revista Educare, 25*(3). https://doi.org/10.46498/reduipb.v25i3.1535

De Jong, P., & Berg, I.K. (2013). *Interviewing for solutions* (4th ed.). Brooks/Cole.

De Shazer, S., Dolan, Y., Korman, H., Trepper, T., McCullom, E., & Berg, I.K. (2007). *More than miracles: The state of the art of Solution-Focused Brief Therapy.* Haworth/Taylor-Routledge.

Dolan, Y. (1991). *Resolving sexual abuse: Solution-Focused therapy and Ericksonian hypnosis for adult survivors.* W.W. Norton & Company.

Fry, W., & Salameh, W. (2004). *El humor y el bienestar en las intervenciones clínicas.* (E. Jáuregui, Trans.). Desclée De Brouwer.

Furman, B. (2013). *Nunca es tarde para tener una infancia feliz: De la adversidad a la resiliencia.* (R. Filella, Trans.). Ediciones Octaedro, S.L.

Furman, B. (2018, 30 May). *Helping clients heal from trauma: Solution-Focused Approach.* Verti. https://verti.se/wp-content/uploads/2017/03/Helping-Clients-Heal-from-Trauma.pdf

Lipchick, E. (2004). *Terapia centrada en soluciones más allá de la técnica. El trabajo con las emociones y la relación terapéutica.* (A. Negrotto, Trans.). Amorrortu editores.

Neipp, M., & Beyebach, M. (2022). The global outcomes of Solution-Focused Brief Therapy: A revision. *The American Journal of Family Therapy*, 1–18. https://doi.org/10.1080/01926187.2022.2069175

Pérez, P. (2006). *Trauma, culpa y duelo: hacia una psicoterapia integradora* (2nd ed.). Desclée De Brouwer.

Pichot, T., & Dolan, Y. (2003). *Solution-Focused Brief Therapy: Its effective use in agency settings.* Routledge.

Pichot, T., & Smock, S. (2009). *Solution-Focused substance abuse treatment.* Routledge.

Superintendencia de Salud (2022, March). *Caracterización de los profesionales de la salud en Chile 2021.* https://supersalud.gob.cl/documentacion/666/articles-20912_recurso_1.pdf

Turnell, A., & Edwards, S. (1999). *Signs of safety: A solution and safety oriented approach to child protection casework.* W.W. Norton & Company.

Vanistendael, S., Gaberan, P., Humbeeck, B., Lecomte, J., Manil, P., & Rouyer, M. (2013). *Resiliencia y humor.* (P. González, Trans.). Gedisa.

Editor reference

Froerer, A., von Cziffra Bergs, J., Kim, J.S., & Connie, E. (2018). Vicarious resilience. In A. Froerer, J. von Cziffra-Bergs, J.S. Kim & E. Connie (Eds.), *Solution-Focused Brief Therapy with clients managing trauma* (pp. 226–235). Oxford University Press.

Chapter 3

In the space between governance and politics

A Solution Focused approach to rethink and operate democratically on public policy

Sofie Geisler (Mexico)

Introduction

I am originally from Greenland and Denmark. Currently, however, I am based in Mexico and work as an adviser and international consultant on change strategies and processes in the Senate of the Republic of Mexico. I see my role as changing political narratives and helping organisations to take action. I have taken the Solution Focused approach and implemented it in large-scale processes such as governance and politics. Over the past decade I have implemented the Solution Focused approach in justice systems, with special emphasis on alternative dispute resolution. This has led to me training more than 1,000 lawyers, public servants, and decision makers in Solution Focused conflict and change management.

Reflect on how your gender influences your work–life and being a Solution Focused practitioner?

"As a woman it must be so difficult to work in that environment", someone said to me, referring to my work in Mexico with decision makers in the public sector and in politics. My first reaction was surprise. "How come?" I asked, and she looked puzzled when she said what she thought to be obvious: "Because you are a woman!"

Of course, I should know what it is like to be a woman in my field of work. However, it struck me that this was not the case. I have never actively related my gender to the many obstacles I constantly face, not even when it is evident that my male colleagues are not dealing with the same obstacles. Thinking about my gender as some kind of determinant has felt like a way of reducing the influence of my own competences, personality, history, and contributions as a *person*, as Sofie, and not as a woman.

In this light, I never question or think of my gender as an explanation or justification. It is never the beginning or the end of any of my arguments. Whatever my situation, I continue asking myself, "What has been working well?", "What would I like to see happen?", and "What can contribute to getting closer to that?" From this perspective, I keep adjusting, adapting, and creating ways to make things

DOI: 10.4324/9781003430254-4

work, without paying much attention to my gender as, for example, the reason why things were and are indeed difficult. This might seem odd when taking into consideration the situation of women in Mexico.

In Mexican society one finds marked differences between men and women, which are reflected in serious labour, social, and economic discrimination. The gender gap is further deepened by a terrifying level of violence, physical and mental mistreatment, and femicides. In 2015–2022, 30 000 women were murdered, which, tragically, broke all kinds of records and placed Mexico among the three countries in the world with the most femicides. For me, as for most women in Mexico, living with my gender is inevitably entangled in a fine web of fear that subtly ties you up and restricts your freedom.

In my work as a Solution Focused consultant in governance and politics, being a woman means dealing on a daily basis with comments on my appearance, hints on how my career could change for the better if I "loosened up a bit", and threats to blacklist me if I do not accept invitations to dinner parties. Frequently, my negotiations on projects suddenly become about what percentage of my salary I should pay to be "protected" from men at work, or the price of "compensation" if I refuse to accept a certain level of intimacy during the contract. In this environment, I have learned that women are seldom supportive or united, but rather fight each other by any means to cut off another's access to attention and privileges. As I experience it in my work, the more the dynamic is dominated by men, the more women become one another's biggest obstacles in their struggle for opportunities.

Recognising that this situation is not related to a particular office or institution, but instead a general cultural dynamic, the question for me has not been whether to give up my work or to fight back, as I will be the first and only one to lose. I have rather focused on how to navigate this environment on a daily basis. Among the many considerations, decisions, and actions to which I pay special attention, several stand out as the most present and useful ones.

First, and perhaps most noticeably, my insistence on not giving in when confronted with the pressure to accept proximity of any kind is supported by my appearance. I am usually perceived as being excessively formal, meaning not only do I dress formally but I also tie back my long hair and come across very formal in informal settings, which makes my behaviour seem ceremonious. This formality is reflected in the manner in which I present my work. Whether it is just a résumé of a meeting or an important presentation for a senator or a president of the High Court, I treat it the same. Though I am frequently questioned about the necessity of this level of formality, it is definitely one of the reasons why I am said to be increasingly respected and "treated differently" than other women.

When finally starting up a project, the process of trust building has just begun. For men in this environment, this often takes place at men-only lunches where they socialise or exchange favours not specifically related to work. For some it also includes sharing moments of leisure such as playing golf or travelling with their partners. As a woman, these options are out of reach, which is why I have to focus more on how to create trust in what I do rather than in who I am. This has led me to change the language in which the Solution Focused approach is commonly communicated among consultants and in books about the practice. In my work, the Solution Focused approach is perceived as a softer, kinder, and more careful technique, which are all characteristics linked to feminine values. For a number of stakeholders, this seems to confirm that the Solution Focused approach is "a nice woman's practice" and that "such an idealistic and gentle take on change cannot be adapted to the harsh reality of governance and politics". I suppose this is said without realising that the implication is that "real" governance is for men, defining a "masculine" perspective.

At first, I tried to use arguments and explanations to show why and how the Solution Focused approach is useful in a macro context. However, explanations are easily conceived as "lecturing", and there is little interest in lessons from a person who happens to be a woman, younger, white, and not even part of the power struggle.

This is one of the main reasons why, years ago, I decided not to describe the Solution Focused approach, its benefits, and how it works, and even stopped mentioning the practice at all. Instead, in every setting, project, and moment, I study how to connect Solution Focused thinking, and often end up simply suggesting "concrete steps" translated into paybacks. And it works!

What started with an obstacle and the need to adapt Solution Focused "language" to a context dominated by masculine and power dynamics has now developed into a way of working that offers interesting opportunities to rethink and rename the Solution Focused approach in practice.

The greater focus and international debate on gender has made me aware that all my years of neglecting the impact of being a woman is indeed part of the culture of inequity that serves to sustain it. In other words, believing that I am solely responsible for the barriers and difficulties I encounter is yet another expression of how gender remains related to structural injustice. However, at the same time it has obliged me to find ways to introduce Solution Focused thinking into environments that appear to be especially closed to the characteristics of the practice – and to women.

What is your good reason for staying a Solution Focused practitioner?

The immediate response to this question is simply that the Solution Focused approach is the most effective way to develop constructive change. It is universal in the sense that it can be used in all cultures and settings. Simultaneously, it is also an amazingly useful guideline in designing, preparing, creating, and continuously improving initiatives for change.

Expanding on this, for me Solution Focused practice is a way of constantly questioning how things are perceived and handled. The anthropological curiosity about what is wanted and what works makes it more likely to recognise opportunities and progress. Nonetheless, what makes it especially useful in my work is the priority Solution Focused thinking places on always seeing people in relation to others. It shows through in many of the questions we use; for example, on how others might notice a certain change, who would be the first ones to see it, and what difference it makes for them.

In governance of public institutions and politics, this interactional view helps to position people at the centre of change. It sounds like a natural thing to do; however, paradoxically, taking the perspective of those people affected by initiatives, laws, programmes, or public policies is often far down the list of considerations. It can even be lost between procedures, spin, and strategies to follow, as well as in the tactics used to address power struggles. The Solution Focused approach is an extraordinary way to bring people back into governance and politics, not as a concept or a box to tick but as real people with needs and hopes for their future.

The fact that Solution Focused practice has its point of departure in what is wanted and looking ahead to the future defines my work. Public policy, programmes, and legislative initiatives are generally created to address a persistent problem from the past that is affecting the present and that must be regulated, avoided in the future, or substituted with something else. Therefore, change is supposed to happen as a consequence of stopping the problem. A detailed vision of the future wanted, or what might be noticed if change happens, is rarely integrated in designing initiatives. This makes it harder to identify signs of progress, connections with other issues, and challenges waiting ahead, which again can lead to costly mistakes with public resources.

And there is more to it. When the process of creating public policies and/or legislation starts with a detailed exploration of the future instead of only relying on a so-called diagnosis of the past, the entire motivation for acting changes. Consider, for example, the difference between, on the one hand, conventional public programmes showing that illiteracy is a problem among significant groups and needs to be resolved and, on the other hand, Solution Focused programmes based on how it would be like if the entire population could share and participate in written communication and what changes could be signs of progress.

In my view, this way of privileging visions of the future in combination with the interactional perspective positions the Solution Focused approach as the missing link between governance or politics and its impact. Changing the way public policy and legislation is generated has the potential to transform the way we face challenges and development, and thus it also holds the seed to transform society.

What would others notice you doing that would tell them that you work from a Solution Focused approach?

- I spend what many find an "unusual amount of time" building a detailed vision of what the future will look like when the change, the project, or the idea is achieved. I suspect that, even for other Solution Focused consultants, I dwell an especially long time on this point.

- I constantly revisit the vision of the future to readjust it and ask myself and the people involved what events, actions, or decisions might bring us closer to that specific situation.
- In most conversations I have on whatever subject needs to be acted on, I will ask how we will know it works as intended and how we will notice the difference. I usually combine this with a systematic exploration of how other people, actors, or sectors are going to notice changes and benefits.
- Though I do not commonly speak directly about Solution Focused practice, it is noticeable that my presentations of projects, results, analysis, speeches, conferences, and proposals for governmental initiatives, state visions, etc. are mostly structured with Solution Focused questions.
- No matter how difficult the situation is, I usually ask what we already have that is working and how it can contribute to us making progress.

Share an exercise that might be useful to other women practitioners

This exercise is for female Solution Focused practitioners (not for our clients):

Imagine what life at work would be like if you could live with your gender the best way possible. Write down at least 15 ways in which you might notice it and what difference it would make. Now imagine that you are going to meet influential legislators of your country. What Solution Focused questions would you ask them to start a change process with the potential to generate what you have visualised?

Share how you adapt the approach and make it your own. Give us five characteristics that are a part of your Solution Focused DNA

What differentiates my "Solution Focused DNA" the most is the integration of "recognition" as a guideline in every moment of my work. For more than 20 years, the core of my practice has been the philosophical idea of recognising what makes humans feel seen as a valuable part of the social world. I believe that the struggle for recognition is what moves most dynamics in society and represents the "grammar of social conflict", to quote Axel Honneth (1996). In my work, recognition is both a tool and a goal because solutions and change are only constructive and possible to maintain if the people involved feel seen as valuable.

In my work, I participate in processes of designing, developing, and coordinating. As such, I am responsible for most steps towards the end results and only do a limited amount of facilitation assignments. Solution Focused practice has become part of every step in my way of working, from my internal dialogue during development to writing, measuring, evaluating, and presenting the results. In this way, part of my Solution Focused DNA is that it is not a tool for certain sessions but rather a way to act and think.

As part of this Solution Focused practice, I often create maps to visualise how change might be noticed among all actors involved or the relevant population groups, as well as what kind of struggle for recognition might be important. These maps often become guidelines for what Solution Focused questions to ask in follow-up.

As well as investing considerable time in creating maps, it is also representative of my practice that I dedicate unusually long periods to exploring a future vision. It is not a question of hours or days but sometimes many weeks.

Finally, I rarely use the concepts, descriptions, and language commonly related to the Solution Focused approach, but find new ways to introduce the practice, adapted to every context. This means that every project has its own "language".

Which female practitioner inspires you and in which way?

I have never before thought of Solution Focused practitioners by virtue of their gender, and it is not an easy task. Inspiration is, for me, a special connection with a person, an environment, atmosphere, or object that makes me see things or act differently. The Solution Focused community is full of such people and connections. Several stand out for me:

- Jenny Clark, for the elegant way in which she simplifies the Solution Focused approach in her practice and introduces the practice as if it is already a natural part of everyday life.
- Carey Glass, for her fascinating ability to connect Solution Focused theory and practice.
- Kati Hankovszky, for her drive and wise innovations.
- Susanne Burgstaller, for taking the Solution Focused approach into new settings, also related to political settings, and with lots of enthusiasm.
- Jocelyne Korman, for an especially caring and thoughtful way of using the Solution Focused approach that always surprises, with results that keep growing.
- Anne-Marie Wulf, for spreading joy and for the energy to keep expanding Solution Focused practice without ever compromising it.

What soft small notion would you encourage other women practitioners to embrace?

I do not know if the notion I share here is soft and small or closer to being big and noisy. However, I would like to encourage others to look upon Solution Focused principles and applications as flexible clues of what works – and not as rules or limitations. Just because Solution Focused practice pays special attention to small signs and changes, it does not imply that it cannot be used in large-scale contexts. And just because the Solution Focused approach has not been introduced in a certain context, it does not mean it is not possible.

For example, there are a growing number of consultants around the world who are using the Solution Focused approach in decision-making, governance, politics, and macro strategies, though it is still perceived by many as almost impossible. We confirm every day that "almost" actually means "plenty of opportunities" that might work. Let's think *with* Solution Focused and not *within* it. There are as many ways to apply a Solution Focused approach as there are people and settings. It can become as big as you want, and there is nothing too big …

My best hopes for other female Solution Focused voices

Imagina que Solution Focused pudiera ser nuestra herramienta para identificar oportunidades que antes no veíamos. Que fuera el instrumento para afinar nuestra mirada de género y poder ver más allá de las barreras que seguimos enfrentando. Imagina que la práctica de Solution Focused nos ayudará a visualizar colectiva-mente cómo sería la sociedad y nuestra cotidianeidad si viviéramos (con) nuestro género de la mejor forma. ¿Será que Solution Focused pudiera ser una manera de generar cambio en el futuro de las mujeres?

Esta es mi esperanza. Imagínate …

Imagine that the Solution Focused approach could be our tool to identify opportun-ities that we didn't see before. That it is an instrument to refine our view on gender and see beyond the barriers that we still face. Imagine that Solution Focused prac-tice helps us visualise together what society and our everyday life could be like if we lived (with) our gender in the best way. Could it be that the Solution Focused approach is actually a way to generate change in the future of women?

This is my hope. Imagine …

Author's reflection

The perception of our gender is largely related to the socio-cultural and economic contexts. It is only one of many influencing factors and not necessarily the most dominant all the time. We might not know what importance it has at the moment or how it varies from one instant to another. When doing work in a rural commu-nity in Mexico, I am not sure which aspects will have the most influence: that I am taller than average; that I belong to a minority of people with white skin, which is easily perceived as belonging to a privileged social class; or that I happen to be a woman.

Writing this chapter has required an effort to focus and isolate gender as a single factor. This has only made it clearer to me how important it is not seeing gender as static but as fluid and in constant change, which also describes my own experience of being a woman. If I had written this contribution last year or were to write it a year from now, it would undoubtedly be different. We should keep this temporality in mind to avoid using gender to create or determine a certain reality in our prac-tice, and instead apply the Solution Focused approach to question which situations or change we want to strengthen. In this way, we move our gaze from how gender influences our practice to how the Solution Focused approach can influence our experience of gender (and the political agenda).

It is part of the essence of doing Solution Focused work – that to which we pay attention tends to grow and become stronger. So, what are we going to talk about next?

Co-constructive editors' reflection

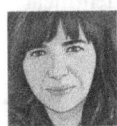 What surprised me about this chapter is that it really talks about gender in a big way and challenges us to think differently.

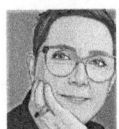 And with a different angle on **doing** Solution Focused practice. Sofie introduces us to her work through a wide description of the environment and the conditions in which she is living and working in Mexico City.

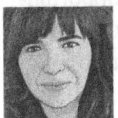 Yes, she shares the vulnerability of being a woman, living with fear, and having limited freedom. Being judged by her gender has influenced her Solution Focused work: instead of promoting it up front, instead of trying to teach people, she has to lead by example.

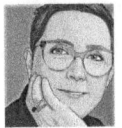 I was paying attention to this as well. These assumptions about women force Sofie to negotiate differently. She constantly has to negotiate about a percentage of her salary and protect herself from not accepting a certain level of intimacy. That is hard to imagine, and it makes good sense that she refers to herself as a person, as Sofie, rather than as a woman.

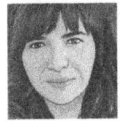 Yes, she describes how hard it is to be a woman in a male-dominated space and how hard it is to be recognised. And you know, what I found amazing is that she says it's about leading by example, it is in her **being** and her **doing** to stay Solution Focused. She, subtly yet consistently, develops and works on change in a Solution Focused way.

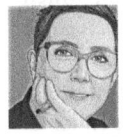 And she's doing it on a larger scale, rather than at those micro levels we have seen described in other chapters. It is great to have these descriptions of how Solution Focused thinking can be adapted into larger scales, and it's also fascinating to imagine how the Solution Focused approach can be used in a changing process of society.

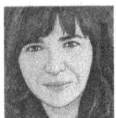 Absolutely. I made a little heart where she wrote, "What is your good reason ...", when she said it brings people back into governance. The Solution Focused mindset makes politics and legislation become more human, and she says it positions people at "the centre of change". That is on a much bigger level, and it is so powerful. This

is what politics and change should look like: constantly **being** a role model, taking discussions back to people, and adding the possibility of future change for people: this is what politics and change should be.

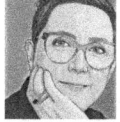

And she's reminding us that it can be different. That it's universal in the sense that it can be used in all cultures and settings.

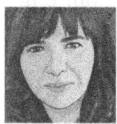

As I was reading that, I was thinking, "Just imagine this can happen in my country". Just imagine, you know. She made me really dream of possibilities everywhere.

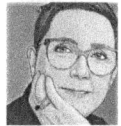

It is nice to be someone who can inspire other people to dream and make changes. I also noticed her interactional view, which changes all the time between people. People are at the centre of change and, although it sounds obvious, we all know that reality is different. There's a difference between intentions, what we wish for, and real life.

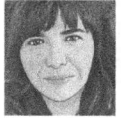

Yes, and then I absolutely loved it when she said that the Solution Focused approach is the "missing link" between governance and politics and their impact. So, what she's saying is that the missing link is talking about and to people and really looking at the impact of possible future change. And I just thought, "Yes, less number talk and more real future visions of possibility and the impact it has on people". And I love that.

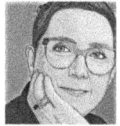

And that brings forward hope, hope that things can be different.

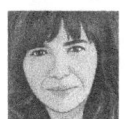

She says recognition is a tool and a goal, which I also love. I like that part of her DNA is that, if we had to look at her internal dialogue, the way she is talking to herself is a Solution Focused conversation. I show it, I do it, I think it, I talk it in my head. I am it.

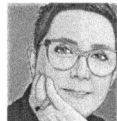

That's a nice way of putting it. I love how her sentences are slightly provocative because it's not said with the intention to provoke. "I do not know if this notion I share is soft and small or closer to being big and noisy." It's like, "Come on, Anne-Marie and Jacqui, what is this about?" Soft, small notion? She is questioning and challenging us, and I appreciate the way she puts it. "I'm in a different context. I'm in a context of politics and governance and I'm going big, doing things on a large scale, so why talk about a soft, small notion?" No, this is big and noisy.

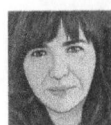

Love that, too. Be big, be noisy. And look for those little clues, and when you hear them, be bold, be big, be noisy about those little things that work, and apply it everywhere. And then she reminds us to think with a Solution Focused lens, let's be it and not keep defending it or teaching it, just be it and be it with a lot of noise.

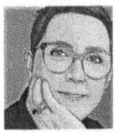

And she invites us to imagine that the Solution Focused approach could be our tool to identify opportunities that we didn't see before. As though it is an instrument to play with, which reminds me of our collection of metaphors. Sofie invites us to redefine our view on gender and see beyond the barriers that we still face. I think it's beautiful.

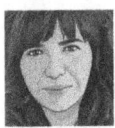

And she challenges us again when she says it is, in part, the essence of **doing** Solution Focused that we need to pay attention to. And I love how she challenges us and in a way says, "Come on girls, what are we gonna talk about next?"

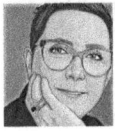

Yes, challenging us to think why the topic of gender is interesting. She is influencing the way you and I think about gender in our practice, and that is really nice. Reminding us that being Solution Focused influences the way we process and co-construct. And then I love that Sofie has no references, because she is not relying on others to **be** Solution Focused; this is her way of **doing** it.

Author reference

Honneth, A. (1996). *The struggle for recognition: The moral grammar of social conflicts.* MIT Press.

Chapter 4

The gift of representation

Solution Focused Brief Therapy as a safe haven for the LGBTQ community

Rebekka Ouer (USA)

Introduction

I am a clinical social worker and supervisor who owns Dallas Rainbow Counseling, a private practice in Dallas, Texas, that has been serving the LGBTQ community since 2011. I have also served as an adjunct professor at the University of Texas at Arlington's School of Social Work, teaching a master's level mental health course. I conduct training on this intersection and have authored *Solution Focused Brief Therapy with the LGBT community: Creating futures through hope and resilience* (Routledge).

Doing this work and being trusted by this community, which is often terribly underserved and whose members are frequently targeted for harassment in our personal and professional lives, is an honour for which I am incredibly grateful. Working in a Solution Focused way with this population has proven to me, more than anything ever could, how powerful, effective, and perfect a fit Solution Focused Brief Therapy is with marginalised communities, and the queer community specifically.

Reflect on how your gender influences your work–life and being a Solution Focused practitioner

In thinking about this answer, I couldn't avoid separating my gender expression from my gender as a woman. My expression has always fallen somewhere on the spectrum between androgynous and masculine. The gendered term I grew up identifying with most was "tomboy", which meant that, as a kid, I dressed, acted, and played more like boys than other girls. As such, I have never expressed myself in very feminine ways, I've never worn dresses or skirts, I don't wear makeup or paint my nails, I've never been romantically or sexually attracted to males, and I knew from a young age that I never wanted to become pregnant or have children.

As a direct result of this, my childhood was riddled with peers and adults making statements like, "You would be so pretty if …" ending that sentence with some more feminine thing I could do to make myself more attractive (seemingly, to the male gaze). That message, in whatever form it came, was frequent, and it was

DOI: 10.4324/9781003430254-5

always loud, clear, and rather annoying. It was, quite simply, that I wasn't doing it right. I wasn't being a girl well enough. As I was – a proudly unapologetic tomboy who would rather shoot hoops and kick a soccer ball in shorts and sneakers than play with Barbies or dress up in cute skirts with a girly hairstyle – I wasn't acceptable. I needed, the world would tell me repeatedly, to soften up and be a better girl.

At this point in my life, as a woman in her 40s, I still sit between androgynous and masculine on that spectrum. I wear pants, sweater vests, and sneakers rather than dresses and high heels, and I am openly gay. The queer community is full of people who, like me, are quite gender diverse in their identities and expressions. As such, it is incredibly important and impactful having therapists as representation for them in the field, seeing some part of themselves in their potential helper, especially in a very conservative state that often shames those who are not heteronormative.

I work with women, men, and non-binary clients who have received some form of shame from our shared world for expressing their gender variance, whether for being too masculine or too feminine, or simply for being transgender and moving towards expressing their gender more authentically. There is an unspoken connection that is invaluable coming from a fellow queer therapist who understands with her whole being, through her own lived experience, what that shame and hurt feels like.

The empathy that lived experience gives me results in a connection that breeds safety from both sides, even before a word is spoken in therapy. As I invite my often gender-diverse clients in, and they in turn see me, wearing pants, Chuck Taylors, and a pullover sweater, they know immediately that I get it. And further, I know that I don't have to worry about them feeling uncomfortable with my gender expression, because of the unspoken understanding that threads this incredible and diverse community together.

That thread is always there, and it's further solidified for my clients when they walk into my office and see a pride flag on my door, and a picture of my wife and me holding hands and sharing our vows on our marriage day. Sometimes I can see clients relax as they see me and then walk into my office space and clock all the signs of safety scattered throughout my décor, informing them that I am not only a safe therapist for them but also a part of this community. They know then that they don't have to spend time educating me about what it is to be queer in this conservative place, with harmful Christo-fascist political pressures bearing down on our existence more and more. That message of safety, often noticed before I speak more than a single sentence to them, is the most impactful foundation with which they can begin this vulnerable relationship.

What is your good reason for staying a Solution Focused practitioner?

I remember learning about Solution Focused Brief Therapy and its core tenets from a professor in college who was also my internship supervisor. He outlined the tenets on a whiteboard during training, and I immediately locked onto the tenet that every client is an expert in their own life. I remember thinking about that and just how much I believed in that incredibly simple yet powerful idea, connecting it to my own life and wishing it were a tenet also valued by our society and culture. To me, that tenet is what makes Solution Focused Brief Therapy a perfect fit with the queer community.

With that tenet as a building block in its foundation, this model of therapy is rooted in empowering our clients to define themselves and their lives for themselves, and trusting them to create their own preferred future on their own terms as their authentic selves. I do not believe there is a more ethical, equitable way to work with marginalised clients in a therapy setting.

What would others notice you doing that would tell them that you work from a Solution Focused approach?

The questions that I ask my clients, whether in the first session or the fifteenth, are rooted in Solution Focused assumptions and tenets. From asking clients about their hope from our work together to asking about their progress since our last visit, from scaling where they are now on a 0–10 range to telling them what I've noticed about their strengths, resources, and talents, every question or statement coming from my therapy room is rooted in Solution Focused Brief Therapy's core tenets and assumptions.

Share an exercise that might be useful to other women practitioners

I often ask a question in-session that involves what one of my incredibly brilliant clients labelled "retrospective analyzation". Sometimes clients come in and believe it is important to tell me about something very difficult that happened to them recently. And rather than refuse because Solution Focused Brief Therapy doesn't care about problems, I do two things: first, I listen carefully as they tell me about the event, and then I ask this:

> Looking back at that very difficult event that you've described, what were some signs that you were moving through that difficulty in a way that was *more* right for you? What would you say you did well to get through it, even though it was challenging?

When I asked my client who coined the term this question, at first she couldn't really answer. (That's when she said, "I don't know, you're asking me to do some retrospective analyzation. I need to think.") So, I patiently waited, and after thinking about it a while through the Solution Focused lens that I had carefully crafted for her, she was able to outline how, in the middle of a panic attack, she was able to care very gently for herself, be patient, remember to breathe and ground herself, drink water and later hot tea, call her best friend for comfort and support, and then take some melatonin so she could get a good night's sleep to put the evening behind her. She remarked after detailing all these things she did so well that she felt very proud of herself for getting through it, a feeling she did not have prior to thinking through and answering that question.

Share how you adapt the approach and make it your own. Give us five characteristics that are a part of your Solution Focused DNA

Compliments for connection: I am and always have been a naturally complimentary person. When I meet someone who has beautiful eyes, or is wearing a cool pair of shoes, or has anything about them that I find striking, I always naturally just mention it, both in my personal and in my work life. So, when I walk out into the lobby to grab a client and bring them back into my office, I will sometimes see something and remark on it. This, I've noticed over the years, serves to put clients at ease very quickly and helps the therapy process move forward more fluidly. This is especially true with teenagers, as I've found it immeasurably helpful in creating space for them to be open to connecting with the process of therapy much more quickly.

Compliments as feedback: as a student years ago who was learning how to become a Solution Focused therapist, I immediately connected with the compliment aspect of the work, and it furthered my belief that this model would fit me perfectly as I continued into my career. And I have found that in doing what Eve Lipchik (2002, p. 153) called "listening with a constructive ear", I am quite naturally able to pick out strengths, resources, values, and hopes from my clients when they are talking about problems. I then offer feedback about what I've learned as I've listened in that Solution Focused way, which can often have a meaningful impact in sessions as clients feel heard, understood, and respected.

Experiments and green flags: specialising in the queer community, I often have teenagers in my office who have come out to their parents as transgender. Their parents are frequently and understandably quite scared about what this might mean for their beloved child, even when their teen is certain they are on the right path by socially transitioning (using a new name, going by different pronouns, and better expressing their gender through clothes and hairstyle). I introduce the parents to the idea of seeing every fully reversible step this teenager takes as an experiment. This means the name, pronouns and gender expression don't have to be seen yet as permanent, rather just as a trial to see if it makes a positive difference. And so, once they take those small, fully reversible steps, I ask everyone to simply notice any green flags along the way that tell them the teen is on the right path. By doing that, by watching out for evidence that they are moving in the right direction, the parents can't help but notice when that evidence begins to appear. Once they have enough evidence for a prolonged period, they are no longer as fearful for their child, who is now happier and more confident because of these steps. The parents are, at that point, eager to do whatever it might take to keep this beloved kid of theirs in that positive mental health space that they often haven't seen in many years. And if, by chance, transition isn't what's right for that teen, that also becomes quite clear. The teen can then recognise that the things they thought they would notice aren't happening and adjust their movements accordingly to move towards their preferred future.

Passion: I have the incredible privilege of feeling as though I am doing exactly what I am supposed to be doing with my life, working here at the intersection of Solution Focused Brief Therapy and the LGBTQ community. With that sense of purpose and fulfilment comes a natural passion for my work and my clients, and that often shows in my office. When clients share their successes with me, such as coming out to loved ones and getting love and support in return, or taking a step towards transition that they were anxious about but are now experiencing the positive effects of, I will celebrate enthusiastically with them in my office. I might high-five a client or say something like, "Wow! How did you do that?" That natural passion is an important aspect of who I am in my work with clients and colleagues.

Resource sharing: one of the things that I also regularly do, and that I believe is important working with the queer community in the American South, is to offer helpful resources that they may not otherwise know about. This includes doctors who are affirming of queer clients, safe and affirming churches in the area, or even books or podcasts about reconciling queerness with religion or coming out at a later age and overcoming one's shame to live authentically. I have a whole lot of helpful resources that I eagerly share at the end of sessions when clients indicate their interest.

Which female practitioner inspires you and in which way?

I feel incredibly lucky to be able to say that my introduction to Solution Focused Brief Therapy came directly from Insoo Kim Berg, back in the summer of 2003. I was a young practitioner invited to a conference where she was the keynote speaker. I had never heard of Solution Focused Brief Therapy, but as I sat in that auditorium and listened to her, and watched videos of her work, I felt as though she was giving me permission to be myself as a fellow social worker. Her presence on that stage as an older woman who had spent her entire career working with people in this unique way, with respect and admiration rather than judgement, shame, or diagnosis, revolutionised the way I began to think about what it could mean to be myself in this field for the rest of my career.

Insoo gave me permission to stop listening to others who worked to convince me that my clients could only be helped through diagnosis, by peeling back the onion of their problems. She showed me that I could trust my instincts and be myself in my work, and so I delved into Solution Focused learning and never looked back. To this day, when I read Insoo's work or watch videos of her sessions, I still feel that important representation as a fellow female social worker who works so passionately and joyfully with her beloved clients. For me, it's a professional kinship unlike any other.

What soft small notion would you encourage other women practitioners to embrace?

One of the lessons I've repeatedly learned from my incredible clients over the years is that discovering and unapologetically honouring your true and authentic self in a world full of others who consistently use varying degrees of shame as a tool to stop you from doing so is the only path to self-love, which, in turn, is the only path to true fulfilment.

So, my notion would be this: as a practitioner, first be authentic to yourself, before applying Solution Focused Brief Therapy or any other therapy model. Then apply the model in a way that aligns best with you as a person, that fits with your values, strengths, passions, and who you naturally are.

My best hopes for other female Solution Focused voices

When you know who you are as a therapist, and you've discovered that Solution Focused Brief Therapy fits best with your integrity and ideals, my very best hope for you (and for your future clients) would be to use those unique-to-you skills and values to work with a community with which you connect the most and about which you feel the most passionate.

I have learned over the past decade just how much representation in the therapy room can be profoundly impactful for marginalised communities. Having queer clients who feel seen, understood, and respected, sometimes even before therapy begins, has been a foundation that makes the rest of therapy much more fluid and successful.

Author's reflection

Working at the intersection of Solution Focused Brief Therapy and the queer community, I have written a book, contributed chapters, and done numerous trainings, but in writing this chapter I realised that I have thought surprisingly little about my gender as it relates to my work and profession. It's been an incredible (and quite challenging) gift to think about these questions.

Writing this chapter and thinking deeply about this has been an invaluable reminder about how representation can be a powerful presence in the therapeutic relationship. I have often said over the years how important representation in media and art can be, but until I thought about these questions I hadn't fully considered how one of life's most impactful and vulnerable relationships – that between a client and their therapist – can be so powerfully affected through the lens of safety and unspoken understanding, by that same representation.

Co-constructive editors' reflection

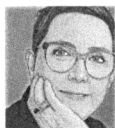

This chapter was really a gift to read. Rebekka shared new knowledge and new information in a context in which I do not ordinarily work and is so different from what I have read before. Rebekka makes it so clear how she uses herself as a representation of the LGBTQ community. I loved that, as you step into her office, the pride flag is there, which is a strong sign to the client who enters the room that she has really thought about how she approaches this community.

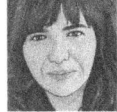

I am getting goosebumps as you speak because for me this chapter was a real gift, a real present. And she writes so often about creating safety and how she owns her role as therapist in creating a safe, accepting space for her clients, where you completely trust the client in every single way to know what is best for them. Rebekka really makes the client the complete expert in every single sense and to me that is complete acceptance.

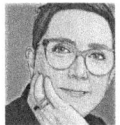

And this is based on her strong values, which she traces right back to her childhood. Her separating her gender expression from her gender as a woman was really interesting and from the beginning she got me to keep reading. She has this passion for people and that is her way of being in life.

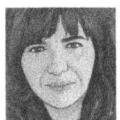

Rebekka reminds us that gender can be fluid and that we cannot assume anything – when we are unsure or in the not-knowing, when you do not know; just ask respectful questions (Ouer, 2016, p. 31) and the client will lead.

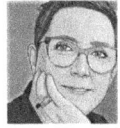

Exactly, and even more curiosity and even more stepping back and stepping back even further and even more not knowing and being made aware of our assumptions; I am so thrilled by this. I got this feeling she's been there herself and is "on the other side", which is even more real for the client, especially when the cultural pressure is so strong.

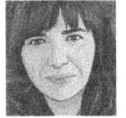

Yes, it felt to me as though Rebekka was giving us her real authentic self in such an honest, truthful way, which allows the client to just be authentic too. And that is the gift, or part of the gift she gives.

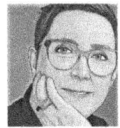

And by doing that she unfolds new worlds, new words, and new perspectives from this stance. And I am so grateful for this because I have really learnt something. She is a strong believer, making strong statements like having a photo of her and her wife holding hands on the wall.

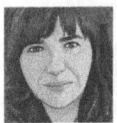

Her strong statements are not done with loud words. She leads from one step behind with visuals and being herself and that is so elegant. And I loved that she saw that in Insoo Kim Berg, who gave her permission to just be herself.

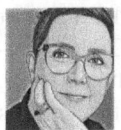

Her description of Insoo is so detailed that it made me feel as though I was right there too, and I loved that she said Insoo gave her permission to trust herself and her instincts in her work. What I really loved was that we all know how to use compliments as feedback, but Rebekka also uses compliments as a way of connecting to the client.

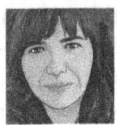

She says, "Compliments make the process move forward and more fluidly", and I love the words she uses because it describes the essence of the Solution Focused approach. The way Rebekka uses and constructs words is so powerful and so beautiful and so mindful. She really made me think on every level, even talking about positive mental health.

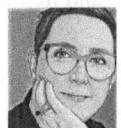

And then I noticed that her way of thinking about resource sharing is different. We don't give advice, we share resources – I love that because it's much more gentle. I will take that with me. I really love that she shares with others, and again it's a gift that she shares not only with her clients but with me as well. She is generous in inviting us into a new understanding. It's like putting a new lens on my Solution Focused camera and seeing something I haven't seen before that I want to use going forward.

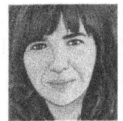

Yes, this lens she is generously sharing with us is all about looking at how we work, how we use language, how we bring ourselves into the session, how we use our intuition, how we accept people, and how we are as therapists. This chapter is about more than just genders – it is about being our authentic self, and she encourages us to honour our true self.

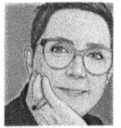

She talks about using your "unique-to-you skills", and this is what makes us true to our authentic self. The role of the therapist is using the Solution Focused approach to show the client the "unique-to-you skills". This is very dynamic and fluid.

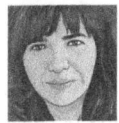

Rebekka is inviting us to use our "unique-to-you' skills as a therapist. Yes, find it in the client but also use your own uniqueness in the sessions. What keeps resonating with me is "Use yourself and your uniqueness" and then add the approach, and do not force the approach on yourself. Make it part of your personal style.

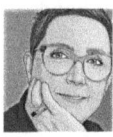

With this approach, you can be you and create your own style. It reminds me we had an EBTA conference called "My Style" and I presented a workshop where I invited everyone to do "silly walks" like in Monty Python, just a silly walk to represent your style and show what your style looks like and that everyone's style is different. You have to find your style.

Author reference

Lipchik, E. (2002). *Beyond technique in Solution Focused therapy: Working with emotions and the therapeutic relationship*. Guilford Press.

Editor reference

Ouer, R. (2016). *Solution Focused Brief Therapy with the LGBT community: Creating future through hope and resilience*. Routledge.

Chapter 5

Finding my own voice

Teri Pichot (USA)

Introduction

I work with some of the most challenging client populations: those struggling with domestic violence, chronic and persistent mental illness, chronic substance misuse, etc. I ran a co-occurring diagnosis treatment centre for over 15 years. It was there that I first fell in love with training professionals to use this mode skilfully with these challenging presenting problems, all within a heavily regulated, problem-focused system. In 2010, I decided to follow my passion for training and developed the Denver Center for Solution Focused Brief Therapy. In addition to working with clients, I now teach internationally, training professionals in what I learned from my Solution Focused mentors.

Reflect on how your gender influences your work–life and being a Solution Focused practitioner

I was raised in the 1970s in California. Although the laws in the United States (US) had been changed to prohibit gender-based discrimination (Quffa, 2016), the gender messages I received growing up were very stereotypical. My father was the sole provider, and my mother stayed at home and raised the children. It was expected that I would marry and become a mother. Any career would be secondary to my husband's and, even then, would most likely be that of a teacher or nurse. I left home and moved to Colorado, where I ultimately followed the expected course of marriage and motherhood.

However, life didn't go according to plan. My daughter died at birth, followed soon after by my marriage, throwing me into a tailspin. What followed was a life-changing exploration of who I am and how this differed from expectations. In my quest to heal my grief, I became a therapist. I never really fit within my family's religious beliefs. While family members seemed to effortlessly live the expected religious life, I could never seem to pray correctly or find the formula to happiness. I always felt like a fraud. I was instead drawn to those who also didn't fit in, who felt lost, judged, and marginalised. Working with those who struggled with substances felt like coming home in many ways.

DOI: 10.4324/9781003430254-6

Working with such an outwardly tough and at times angry or anti-authoritarian population was a challenge. In the 1980s–1990s, addiction counsellors were primarily men and oftentimes those who were recovering themselves. I was neither. I was young and a woman, and I didn't appear to belong. The treatment model was confrontational, and I was expected to address denial and cognitive distortions in my clients. I had to find another way to connect with them. Motivational Interviewing came along and seemed more promising; however, it was ultimately just a gentler way to confront the addictive behaviour. When Charlie Johnson and Jeff Goldman (1998) introduced me to Solution Focused Brief Therapy and eventually to Insoo Kim Berg and Steve de Shazer, I knew I had found the answer. It was a model that was genuinely respectful and curiosity-based. This was a model through which I knew I could be myself and find the heart of the most angry and distraught human being.

So how does this fit with my gender? Solution Focused practice allows me to focus on connecting with people, to hear and respect whomever I meet regardless of my stature or past experience. There's no need to verbally overpower, outmanoeuvre, or wear a person down. There's no pathological puzzle to be solved. No need for intimidation or posturing. It is about connecting with each unique person in a genuine and meaningful way.

What is your good reason for staying a Solution Focused practitioner?

It is commonplace to make assumptions, and many of those assumptions presuppose the worst about others. When we make assumptions, we are no longer seeing the unique person in front of us. When we step into a knowing stance, we are no longer curious. I find this way of interacting with others exhausting.

In Solution Focused Brief Therapy we assume the best about people and take people at face value. De Shazer et al. (2007) referred to this as staying on the surface, and said, "Don't think. But observe" (p. 101). We seek to stay in the "not-knowing" stance (Pichot with Smock, 2009, pp. 46–47). This results in us becoming curious in the absence of information. This way of thinking is much less likely to lead to misunderstandings.

Throughout my career I have worked alongside professionals who used bullying, intimidation, belittling, and veiled threats with colleagues. There would be a competitive tone as they touted their accomplishments. They worked from the deficit-based either/or stance. In Solution Focused practice we work from a cooperative yes/and stance. We can both succeed. As Kenneth Gergen (2009) states, even during apparent disagreement, we can have and honour multiple perspectives.

This is the way of working and thinking in the world that gives me energy and joy. This is true to who I am and what I believe. It is a cooperative, curious stance, both with clients and with professionals and colleagues alike. While I don't always succeed in my ideals and live what I believe, it challenges me to do better, to be better. It makes me a better human and, in turn, empowers me to better partner with those around me.

What would others notice you doing that would tell them that you work from a Solution Focused approach?

There are three main ways someone can identify that I am working in a Solution Focused way. The first is that I strive to set aside jargon, labels, and assumptions as much as possible. Not only do I do my best not to use jargon and labels, but I also make an effort to not think in those terms. What we think influences what we ask our clients and our ability to truly listen to them (Pichot with Smock, 2009, p. 50). This is true about diagnostic labels as well as socially acceptable labels such as "recovery", "self-esteem", "happy", etc. When we allow ourselves to use even these gentler labels, we tend to forget we have no idea what the person is talking about. Instead, I have them describe what this looks like. This description is much more meaningful in my work.

The second way people can tell I'm Solution Focused is in what I attend to during conversations (Korman et al., 2013). When working in a Solution Focused way, I listen for what the client wants, what is working, and what is important to them. These are the areas I explore. I listen with great compassion when clients talk about problems, yet I don't ask questions. This isn't where change lies. I purposefully use the client's exact words to gently tap the conversation in a helpful direction. It's a powerful way of talking with clients.

The last way people can tell I am using Solution Focused practice is the assumption of good intent. Insoo Kim Berg (personal communication, 1994) used to say, "You must have a good reason" when working with clients who talked about behaviours that were seemingly inappropriate. I learned from her to set aside judgement and trust that clients' behaviour makes sense within the context of their lives. It's important to understand that this does not excuse bad behaviour, but it does help us to better respond from a place of empathy and compassion. Learning to step into the client's world to explore their good reasons is at the heart of both responding with compassion and genuinely seeing the good in people.

Share an exercise that might be useful to other women practitioners

A helpful thing is the use of a recording device. Start by simply recording a professional conversation (with a consenting client, coworker, professional colleague, or even just yourself talking about a case). When listening to the recording, listen carefully for moments in the conversation where your words indicate curiosity and not-knowing. Notice what difference this makes to the person's response. Also, listen carefully for subtle language clues that imply opinion or bias. Explore how you would speak differently if you instead returned to that curious stance.

Share how you adapt the approach and make it your own. Give us five characteristics that are a part of your Solution Focused DNA

Integration of therapy dogs: one of the most common topics professionals ask me to address is my inclusion of therapy dogs in my work (Pichot, 2012). While it's a very small part of my work, it's one that often stands out as the most unusual and engaging. I have had dogs for over half a century, and I cannot imagine life without their companionship and love. When I was training my first rough-coat collie, Rockefeller, I noticed how many people approached me to talk about the dog who normally would never have engaged. Spontaneous conversations about difficult subjects were initiated by strangers. Parents actively followed my directions to ensure that children acted safely. They were eager to explore how best to work with their children to get the desired result. Others disclosed very painful pasts, and readily explored hopes for the future. Somehow, in the presence of a dog, all these risk-taking behaviours occurred without any effort. These conversations were the kind we struggled to create with clients in the challenging environment of a treatment programme.

And, so, the idea was formed to train Rockefeller as a therapy dog and include him in my work. I remember speaking to Insoo and being nervous about how she might respond to the idea of me adding a dog into the model that she and Steve de Shazer loved so much. During a walk together, I carefully introduced the subject. I stared at the ground nervously, waiting for her to dismiss the idea as trivial. To my surprise, she said, "I have a grand dog. I can see how they would be good at Solution Focused therapy."

For over ten years, Rockefeller worked with clients and staff. He demonstrated how small steps such as a tail wag, a gentle lick, or a snuggle could make big changes in the environment and in the people around him. He was the subject of many Relationship Questions and created many exceptions during client sessions. Other therapy dogs have come after him, but none could ever fill his paws. He will always have a special place in my heart for the lessons he taught about how animals can partner with us in our Solution Focused work.

Living a Solution Focused life: Yvonne Dolan and I wrote about the three stages of becoming a Solution Focused therapist (2003, p. 11). We explained that many people use Solution Focused practice only in the initial two stages. The first stage is when one takes Solution Focused tools, such as the Miracle Question or Scaling, and uses them in a problem-focused context. When used in this way, problems continue to be the focus of treatment. The second stage is when one takes the Solution Focused tools as well as the Solution Focused way of thinking and uses both with clients. In this stage, Solution Focused work is just something to do within the context of a client session.

In the third stage, the professional not only adopts the Solution Focused tools and way of thinking in working with clients but also seeks to bring this way of thinking into their work with colleagues and into their personal life. It becomes transformational. When conflict arises, they become curious and assume the best about the other's intentions. They seek to refrain from "us vs them thinking" and instead move into a space of collaboration and yes/and. When seeking to live a Solution Focused life, one does not "arrive". It's a commitment and a process of self-awareness and improvement. It's a way of thinking about other people and a language used when working with any person in any setting.

Solution Focused group work: most substance misuse treatment is done in the context of groups. While there had been some writing about Solution Focused groups in the 1990s, most of this was in the context of the first stage of incorporating Solution-Focused practice into the work. They took some of the tools, such as Exceptions, Scales, and Strengths, and used them in the context of traditional problem-focused group practice. We were the first to use and later write about how to completely rethink group modality to fully integrate not only the Solution Focused tools but also the way of thinking (Pichot & Dolan, 2003; Pichot with Smock, 2009). For example, problem-focused groups encourage people to actively give advice/suggestions to other members. This directly contradicts the Solution Focused principle, "The solution is not necessarily directly related to the problem" (Pichot & Dolan, 2003, p. 13). In Solution Focused practice, similar problems don't mean similar solutions; therefore it doesn't make sense for one member to give advice to another. In addition, many of the clients' initial problems stemmed from taking advice from others. I don't want clients to give each other advice/suggestions. Instead, I want to create an environment in which clients think independently about their own desired futures and identify their own unique solutions. There's a significant benefit in inviting clients to explore their solutions in a setting in which others in the group might have a completely different solution. This helps clients to develop confidence in their solutions and protects them from peer influence. This different way of working means that the facilitator, like a traffic cop, ensures everyone safely clears the intersection on their way to their desired destination rather than being the passive facilitator of a group discussion.

I am not looking for strengths or resources: a common way of describing Solution Focused practice is as a strength-based model. While that's correct on an academic level (where models are classified as either deficit-based or strength-based), I don't find that way of sorting helpful on a practical learning/application level. This is something I learned from Steve de Shazer (personal communication, 7 January 2004). Regarding the use of the word "strengths" and the concept of looking for "strengths", Steve said, " 'Strength' is an interpretation and a generalisation that accidentally hides details that might be usefully highlighted." The concept of looking for strengths and resources results in us moving back into an expert-based stance, which requires labels and assumptions. Instead, we are looking for what is working as defined by the client (Pichot & Dolan, 2003, p. 13). Solution Focused practice can best be described on a practice level as an efficacy-based model.

When professionals are in the mindset of looking for client resources, they shift back into the expert-based stance of problem-solving. They start to believe that past resources might be helpful now or in the future. They then make suggestions and assert their well-intentioned agenda of moving past exceptions and resources into the future to solve the presenting problem. In Solution Focused practice we notice past successes. When we do this from a genuinely curious stance, the client will naturally determine what might be helpful in the future. It's a subtle and powerful shift.

Which female practitioner inspires you and in which way?

It was Insoo Kim Berg who inspired me to become the Solution Focused practitioner I am today. I first met her in 1995, when she and Steve visited the Friday night team in Colorado. The team was a small group of therapists who worked with a one-way mirror using Solution Focused Brief Therapy with couples experiencing domestic violence. Insoo was invited to work directly with the clients, and her way of working with the couple can best be described as a "presence". She was empathic, yet she was clearly, purposefully guiding the conversation. I took every opportunity to learn from Insoo. She asked about my work, and I shared my challenges leading a Solution Focused team through a highly regulated, problem-focused culture. At times I would reach out to Insoo in tears as the Solution Focused model and my leadership were challenged and regulators and colleagues made it clear that Solution Focused Brief Therapy didn't meet their idea of standard of care. In my darkest times, she would say, "They need you! Where will these clients go if you and your team don't get through this?"

It was Insoo's ability to credibly speak about and use Solution Focused practice in settings in which she was challenged that inspired me the most. She didn't defend. She would simply say, "That's one way to see it, and there's another". When professionals insisted that the only ethical intervention would be to explore the client's pathology, she would respond, "That could work. What are you hoping will be different?" Her gentle spirit disarmed the harshest critic, and yet her persistence and passion for the model were unmatched. I sat at Insoo's home and listened late into the night as she passionately spoke about clients and a different way to work with them. I never heard her say an unkind word about a client. Never a hint of burnout – just passion and belief in people. She taught me to think and live in a Solution Focused way. This was not a model that was just for client sessions. It was a stance and a way of thinking about all people.

I will never forget her smile, her kind tone, and her gentle support and compassion. She took me under her professional wing, for which I will always be grateful. She gave me courage to find my professional voice, reminding me it is possible, and that I am doing this for the clients.

What soft small notion would you encourage other women practitioners to embrace?

My hope is that other women will truly embrace that this model is not just for clients but is instead a way of thinking about people.

My best hopes for other female Solution Focused voices

My best hope for other female voices is that they find their unique vocal depth, tone, and quality. I hope they stay strong and true to themselves without falling prey to the misperception that louder, different, or bigger is better. Each voice is perfect and valued.

Author's reflection

We all are given a choice. We can either assume that experienced hardship is the result of discrimination and due to factors outside our control (which may, in fact, be true) and respond with defensiveness or pain, or we can view these aspects as simply part of who we are and therefore focus on moving forward to integrate our experiences into our desired future. I can't know for sure if my softer style is because I am a woman, or if the harsher style of my past colleagues was because they were men. I'm not sure it truly matters. What matters is that I have found my voice, one that is consistent with who I am and one I can use in a genuine way to make a difference in this world.

Co-constructive editors' reflection

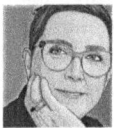

It is amazing. I can already see after reading four or five chapters that almost everybody starts by going back to the past. It's interesting to realise that when talking about the present, we go back to the past to introduce our background and the way in which we were raised to say a bit about how things are today.

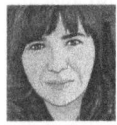

Anne-Marie, that reminds me about what you and I wrote in Chapter 1. We said being, doing, and then the context of time. And it's as if everybody goes back to that context of time.

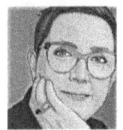

Yes, they define their DNA from when they were born. We are invited into different contexts, different families, different lives, and, even though we are not that far apart from each other in terms of age, we are still invited into so many different contexts. That is really fascinating.

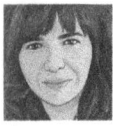

And Teri positions her context so clearly in her time frame, and then she links that to her good reason for being a Solution Focused practitioner.

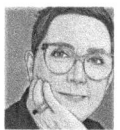

And she shares with us her cultural background and I realised that there's a lot embedded in her DNA. It became clear to me when she wrote about being raised in a very religious family. I was struck by this sentence: "a life-changing exploration of who I am and how this differed from expectations". Other people's expectations of us, our parents' or siblings' expectations, are not what we necessarily become.

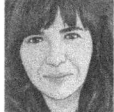

Yes, that was beautiful. Because it also makes me think, this is the journey we go on with ourselves and our clients. And then what also stood out for me, that I personally really appreciated, is that she kept referring to there being no pathological puzzle to solve. And then, later on, she says she does not "do labels" and does not "get caught up in the jargon". So, her way of **doing** Solution Focused and her belief about her clients is that she doesn't have to solve any pathological puzzle and that she's not going to label anybody.

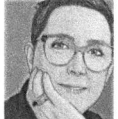

And I think that is a Solution Focused stance very close to Steve de Shazer's heart. Also, stating that, for her, the Solution Focused approach is not strength-based and she does not look for strengths and competencies. And I understand what she means.

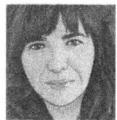

Anne-Marie, this bit me on the nose too; she says it's not strength-based but rather searching for what works. I found that very, very interesting and wow …

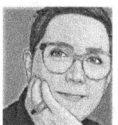

And looking for strengths and resources could lead us back into an expert-based stance. However, this makes me think that maybe it's not either/or, but both/and. Maybe we can talk about strengths depending on how we talk about it.

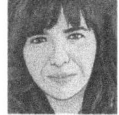

I totally agree with what you've just said; that piece also struck me. And I too made a note here that maybe it can be both. Maybe it can be a strength-based way of looking at people and looking for what is going right, but it does depend on the language which you use to reflect the strength or the compliment or the "what has worked".

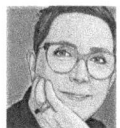

I think it's in the process. I like to ask a child, "What does it require from you to do your homework?" and he might respond, "I need to be focused, I need to concentrate, or I need to ask a classmate". I then follow up with, "So, what would you call someone who can do that?" And then the description of the competences and strengths comes from the client himself. That's not my values, but using the words that the clients use to describe their lives.

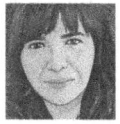

For me, when we do that, we are helping the client re-remember or sometimes even realise their own strength in their own words. I find searching for strengths very valuable and I do it all the time. What

I would like to add a lot more of is what Teri is teaching me, and that is to search more for everything that is working. The other thing I really liked that she highlighted is that she looks for the good reasons, because it takes away all judgement. And I love that.

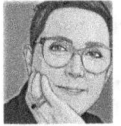

And it allows us to stay in a curious, not-knowing position. When we accept that there has to be good reasons, the next step to follow is to explore what those good reasons are. You have good reasons, otherwise you wouldn't have done it, which doesn't necessarily mean that I have to think it's a good reason too, because it's your good reasons.

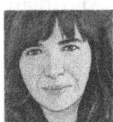

And that links to what you said about that not-knowing and the curiosity stance with which we enter the space.

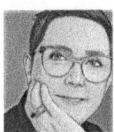

Exactly, which is so important. It also reminds me of when Teri writes about this labelling that you talked about. We do not only not-label clients in the sense of a diagnostic way; we also don't have assumptions about their behaviour. When you see a person laughing, you could assume he's happy, but we don't – instead we ask.

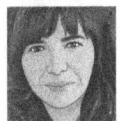

Yes. To be constantly curious even about constructs such as recovery or confidence. What does recovery look like for you? How would you show that you are recovering? Teri doesn't make any assumptions on what that looks like. She will ask somebody.

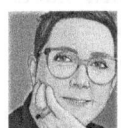

I was training social workers this week in how to talk with children and I heard one participant ask another, "What does busy look like to you?" and I was so pleased, because that was a good question. It is stepping back, and even more not-knowing.

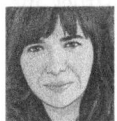

Reading this chapter made me realise that our work is all about stepping back. And then stepping back again.

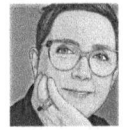

Exactly. It's a stepping back again. Okay, I know I need to take one step back, but then when I am there, I take another step back.

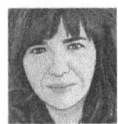

And then something that also came out for me was how she wrote that she is purposefully helping people transform and guide, purposefully guiding the conversation. So, it's stepping back and stepping back again in order to purposefully guide the conversation in the direction that the client wants. It's not just stepping back and leaving it. It's stepping back to purposefully guide the conversation to what is most important to the client and who the client really is. And it reminds me of the concept of not-knowing and leading from one step behind. I also loved how Teri has adapted and integrated dogs into the approach.

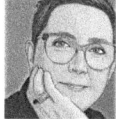 Making it her own and finding new ways that made sense to her. I also thought it was so interesting to read about the three stages that she and Yvonne Dolan talked about. The first stage is to integrate the techniques, the second stage is to use the techniques and the tools with your client, and, finally, in the third stage to not only use the approach in your professional life but also embed it in your veins, which I think is a way of living, and definitely part of Teri's DNA.

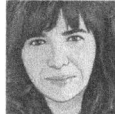 And I love when she says it becomes transformational. It transforms you and then it doesn't just become a technique we're applying with our clients; it becomes a way of living our lives. What else stood out for me was what she wrote about Insoo Kim Berg, because Teri had this wonderful personal journey with Insoo. I loved how Insoo just gently said, "Well, that's one way and there's another way" and how she just stuck to her beliefs and didn't defend the approach, but just stuck to it. Loved that.

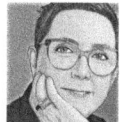 Yes, which I think can be difficult when you're doing training. Just to go with, "that's one way of seeing it and that's another".

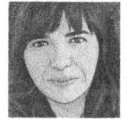 Especially if you're training in organisations or settings where the problem model or medical model is so strongly put in the foreground. But we don't have to defend it. We just have to say, well that's one way, here's another.

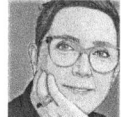 Such beautiful memories arising of Insoo in this chapter. It reminds me that Teri isn't the only or the first one to mention Insoo Kim Berg. Several of our authors talk about Insoo as the person who has influenced them the most, and I think this might also turn out to be a kind of a memorial to Insoo. Never thought about that, but she has had an impact on so many people and for me it is a bit of gratitude and gratefulness. Teri remembers these special moments with Insoo and shares them with us. I only had the opportunity to see Insoo once, yet her presence and impact on people was remarkable. I think it is just such a treasure to have these recollections shared by Teri, really special and so beautiful. "She gave me courage to find my professional voice" – how beautiful is that?

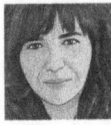 Insoo gave us all a kind of permission to just do it in our own way and to be true to yourself. I am so grateful to Teri for sharing her relationship with Insoo with us and for Inoo for being like the mother figure who says, "Of course, go for it, make it your own". Beautiful chapter. Very beautiful. Very helpful.

Author references

De Shazer, S., Dolan, Y., Korman, H., Trepper, T., McCollum, E., & Berg, I.K. (2007). *More than miracles: The state of the art of Solution-Focused Brief Therapy.* Haworth.

Gergen, K.J. (2009). *Relational being: Beyond self and community.* Oxford University Press.

Johnson, C.E., & Goldman, J. (1998). A Solution-Focused approach to safety in cases of domestic violence. In M.F. Hoyt (Ed.), *Constructive therapies 2: Volume 2* (pp. 184–196). Guilford Press.

Korman, H., Beavin Bavelas, J., & De Jong, P. (2013). Microanalysis of formulations in Solution-Focused Brief Therapy, Cognitive Behavioral Therapy, and Motivational Interviewing. *Journal of Systemic Therapies, 32*(3), 31–45.

Pichot, T. (2012). *Animal assisted Brief Therapy: A Solution-Focused approach* (2nd ed.). Taylor and Francis.

Pichot, T., & Dolan, Y. (2003). *Solution-Focused Brief Therapy: Its effective use in agency settings.* Haworth.

Pichot, T., with Smock, S.A. (2009). *Solution-Focused substance abuse treatment.* Routledge.

Quffa, W.A. (2016, December). A review of the history of gender equality in the United States of America. *Social Sciences and Education Research Review, 3*(2), 143–149.

Chapter 6

Solution Focused Single Session Therapy

Small conversations for big social change

Alesya Courtnage (Canada)

Introduction

I began my career as a mental health practitioner in 2001 with an education obtained from an American university that was steeped in the traditions of psycho-dynamic theories. I was told to memorise the Diagnostic and Statistical Manual of Mental Disorders and trained in mental health status exams and risk assess-ments. I was taught that "big" problems required big therapy – meaning long-term, intensive, and insight-oriented. When I returned to Canada and began working in a child and family agency I carried these teachings with me, naively confident in my ability to make a difference in a public sector system that had the best interests of the community at heart. I found Solution Focused Brief Therapy in 2008, at a time when I felt burnt out and frustrated with the inefficiencies and inequities of Canada's publicly funded mental healthcare system. In 2008, I attended my first workshop in Solution Focused Brief Therapy and fell in love with the hope, opti-mism, and respect that drive this way of working with others. Currently, Ontario is a wellspring of mental health walk-in clinics and my clinical work in Solution Focused Single Session Therapy (SF-SST) has inspired me to continuously explore the potential of SF-SST both as a service delivery model and as an effective clinical intervention. This passion has allowed me to lead and attend trainings in SF-SST around the world.

Reflect on how your gender influences your work–life and being a Solution Focused practitioner

In the early days of my career as a psychotherapist I worked at a publicly funded, community-based, child and family mental health agency in Toronto, Canada. With three children under the age of five I felt exhausted in my role as a mother and frus-trated with my inability to engage fully with the profession for which I had trained. I felt guilty about leaving my children to go to work, and guilty about leaving work to care for my children.

Additionally, I was disillusioned, working in a system and environment that was not meeting the needs of the children and families that we claimed to support. The

DOI: 10.4324/9781003430254-7

traditional mental health service delivery model consisted of a series of assessment meetings (up to six), followed by a treatment planning meeting, then an indefinite number of weekly therapy sessions. Sessions were almost always offered during the day, requiring parents to take time off from work to attend sessions with their children. Many of the children and families I worked with were from marginalised communities. A large proportion of the families were headed by single mothers. With limited resources available to them, entire families relied on public transportation to travel to and from therapy appointments, thereby extending the amount of time required to attend sessions. With very few exceptions, mothers bore the responsibility of talking to professionals, managing school-related issues, setting up appointments, and bringing children to appointments. I attended countless meetings with women who expressed being overwhelmed by and frustrated with the demands of the system around them, and the judgement that surrounded non-compliance. With my own identity as a mother in the early stages of development, I felt a profound sense of despair at colluding with a system that made it almost impossible for people in general, but women in particular, to feel competent and capable.

In 2011, as part of a city-wide initiative, the agency where I worked was asked to establish a mental health walk-in clinic (MH-WIC) in order to address the debilitating waitlist for services. The philosophy of MH-WICs is dramatically different from traditional constructs of mental health service delivery. The MH-WIC does not require assessment, diagnosis, or referral. In many MH-WIC models there is no pre-screening or criteria for service. Whoever walks in is guaranteed service (Slive & Bobele, 2012). There is no commitment to additional services and individuals are seen by a mental health professional the same day that they seek help (Slive & Bobele, 2011).

A number of years prior to this I had trained in Solution Focused Brief Therapy. Unlike many of my colleagues, who resisted the ultra-brief format of this work, I felt that I was presented with an opportunity to practise clinically in a way that was congruent with my personal epistemology and value system. At that time, my agency's MH-WIC was located in the basement of a Chinese grocery store in a shopping mall in the North Etobicoke community of Toronto, Ontario. The community was characterised by ethnic and racial diversity and home to many new Canadian settlers. It was during this period that I became more and more interested not only in *what* was happening in sessions but also in *how* people were getting into the sessions themselves.

The agency became a natural stopping point for members of the community. Families arrived for sessions after stressful shopping upstairs, teenagers were escorted by best friends after a heart-to-heart in the coffee shop, and parents promised sweets from the bakery in exchange for attending a session. Due to the many languages and levels of English literacy represented within the community, the intake process was kept to the bare minimum. For the first time in my career, I was seeing clients who were experiencing problems, both big and small, in real time. Accessing support for a bad day at school was no more or less difficult than accessing support for an assault. Within months of opening, the MH-WIC had expanded from one evening to four and the agency was serving more clients than ever before. Solution Focused Brief Therapy, with its foundational principle of treating every session as though it were the first and last, was a natural fit.

This experience impacted me greatly. Long before, I had noticed that within the broad field of psychotherapy there was much discussion about the clinical models used in therapy sessions and far less discussion about models that support service users' access to support. While many would argue that clinical models and service delivery models are separate and distinct, my personal experience is that the ease with which service users are able to access services often influence clinical outcomes. In my experience, the practice of SF-SST alleviates a significant amount of stress, as it does not call for weekly scheduled meetings, something that I, as a mother of three children, would have found very difficult to manage.

What is your good reason for staying a Solution Focused practitioner?

Throughout my career I have received messages that a service user's willingness to "engage" in therapy over a period of time was a sign of success. When service users missed, cancelled, or rescheduled appointments, they were often labelled "resistant" or "not ready for change". Their files would be closed, resulting in denied access to services. However, in my experience, service users' difficulties attending appointments have little to do with their desire for change and are instead the consequence of systemic barriers connected to accessing services.

I believe strongly that mental health systems need to be cost-efficient, accessible, responsive, and sensitive to the complex needs of people challenged with mental health difficulties. The dominant hegemonic medical model proposes that early assessment and diagnosis is an essential component of mental health treatment. However, this approach requires people to participate in lengthy assessments prior to receiving mental health intervention. Additionally, scheduling and attending assessments compound the delay in receiving service and therefore do not address the issue of expedient access. Within this context, SF-SST, often located within MH-WICs, has emerged as the first point of contact for many people seeking quick access to mental health support (Cait et al., 2017). Given that the premise of SF-SST calls into question the necessity and clinical helpfulness of assessment-based, medical model approaches, it is my position that the continued presence and expansion of Solution Focused Brief Therapy represents a disruption to the patriarchal, medical model approach to service delivery that has contributed to the worsening mental health of service users over time. Therefore, my best good reason for continuing to practise SF-SST is that I believe that it has the ability to effect change at both micro- and macro-system levels.

What would others notice you doing that would tell them that you work from a Solution Focused approach?

I believe that the strongest influence of SF-SST has shown up in my parenting. Over the years, one of my primary motivators for practising SF-SST has been the mothers I have met throughout my career who are doing the best they can to balance the demands of work, family, and personal life. In raising a family of my own, I hope that I have transferred some of the resilience and optimism that I have learned from my service users to my children. I hope my parenting has reflected my belief that obstacles can be overcome and that life holds an infinite number of possibilities.

Share an exercise that might be useful to other women practitioners

Like many Solution Focused practitioners, I view hope as a powerful agent of change and as an important, if not essential, component of all therapeutic conversations. In recent years, I have been fortunate to learn about Hope Theory, a theoretical model first conceptualised by Charles Snyder (2002). Using Snyder's Hope Theory as a basis, I have developed a cross-theoretical framework that drives my SF-SST practice. Hope Theory posits that all change begins with the identification of an outcome, and this aligns well with the Solution Focused practice of beginning sessions by asking the question, "What are your best hopes from us talking today?" Interestingly, Snyder (2002) identifies that, in the process of both establishing and pursuing an outcome, people often engage in an appraisal of outcome value. According to him, people who experience high levels of hopeful thinking naturally "check back" on their desired outcomes to ensure that the potential value of the outcome is worth the cognitive and behavioural effort that will be required to attain the outcome. When people check back and affirm their desire for an outcome, it creates a motivational feedback loop that drives the pursuit of their outcomes and makes them more likely to overcome potential obstacles that may impede the attainment of the outcome. Snyder believes that this positive feedback loop is especially important in the "getting started stage", which tends to occur before people take action to attain their desired outcome. As people often seek out mental health support as a first step towards change, it would seem timely to purposefully cultivate the benefits of the appraisal process.

"Appraisal Question" exercise

Given this, in my practice I have begun to develop and incorporate a category of questions that I refer to as Appraisal Questions. These are questions whose intention is to invite the client into a moment of reflection on whether the outcome that they initially identified is something that they still believe is worth the effort of pursuing. These questions serve the function of growing the level of desire for the outcome. Essentially, the more a person wants something, the more likely they are to figure out a way to get it. Examples of Appraisal Questions that can be used throughout the session include:

- *Is that good for you?*
- *What will you notice about yourself that tells you this is right for you?*
- *What tells you that this is worth it?*

Share how you adapt the approach and make it your own. Give us five characteristics that are a part of your Solution Focused DNA

I believe that my Solution Focused DNA has developed into two separate strands over time. The first is located in the broad system of mental health service delivery, the second in the intimate space of therapy sessions.

Macro-level Solution Focused DNA

Solution Focused Single Sessions contribute to social justice: I have long questioned both the necessity and effectiveness of the patriarchal hegemonic orientation towards clinical practice that requires long-term therapy for all. Many clients with whom I have worked have been systemically marginalised and do not have the ability to conform to the demands of traditional, weekly, ongoing therapy. I believe strongly that in order to create an equitable, accessible, and effective mental health system, we must include policies, practices, and service delivery models that question the taken-for-granted assumptions of the Euro-Western medical model conception of mental healthcare.

The existence of SF-SST is an intervention in and of itself: By definition, SF-SST is flexible and responsive to the needs of the service user, as SF-SST offers them opportunities to receive service at times that work best for them. The idea that a person can be presented with options to self-determine the frequency and intensity of their mental health treatment is a radically different approach to the expert-driven medical model that has defined mental health service delivery for over a century.

Micro-level Solution Focused DNA

My micro-level Solution Focused DNA has three characteristics, each of which corresponds to one component of Hope Theory, and which represents one phase of an SF-SST session. Guided by the idea that human actions are driven by the desire to fulfil goals, Snyder (2002) defined hope as "the perceived capability to derive pathways to desired goals, and motivate oneself via agency thinking to use those pathways". Snyder's Hope Theory posits that hope is a cognitive state that occurs as a result of the interplay between goals (the mental target), pathways (routes to the goal), and agency (the perceived ability to attain the goal). Snyder theorised that once a goal is identified and established, a continuous back-and-forth occurs between pathways and agentic thinking. Pathways and agency thoughts are both iterative and additive. As a result, people with high levels of hope will experience fluidity and flexibility in the development of routes towards their goals.

Phase 1 – hope identification (goals): the first task of every SF-SST session is to identify what the client wants from the session. While this is common practice for many Solution Focused practitioners, Hope Theory allows us to understand that the identification of what people want, commonly known as the "best hope", is the necessary starting point of all change. Not only is it the primary building block of hope, but Snyder (1994) also says that the desire to attain goals is one of the primary driving forces behind human action. As such, the identification of the best hope is essential to effective SF-SST.

Phase 2 – hope activation (agency): the second task of every SF-SST session is to ask questions that invite people to describe themselves from a position of capacity. In Hope Theory, if a person is having difficulty attaining their goals, it is most likely due to struggles around agency, or a person's belief in their ability to attain their goals. Solution Focused questions that elicit internal resources and capacities offer service users an opportunity to reconstruct themselves through the lens of their hoped-for futures.

Phase 3 – hope empowerment (pathways): the final task of every SF-SST session is to get out of the way of your service user. Hope Theory posits that all three components of the theory work together iteratively to increase hopeful thinking, meaning that if you impact one component, you can impact them all. It is my belief that the ways in which people decide to achieve their best hopes are for them to decide and perform outside of the therapy sessions. Meaningful behaviour change must occur in the real world, not in the controlled setting of a therapy session. As such, it is my belief that the best use of time in SF-SST is spent on growing desire for a person's best hope and increasing their belief in their capacity to achieve the thing they want most.

Which female practitioner inspires you and in which way?

I have likely not met the female practitioner who inspires me the most because she is too busy and overwhelmed attempting to balance her home and work life. She has likely not attended a conference because she doesn't want to leave her children at home. She has not written a book because she is exhausted at the end of the day and has no energy left to think. She is doing the best that she can to care for the people she loves the most, all while balancing an impossible caseload in a broken system.

The female practitioner who most inspires me is she who goes unnoticed. In spite of all of the challenges, she displays grace, humility, and compassion throughout her practice and her life. The female practitioner I admire the most does not seek the spotlight. She may be undervalued by her colleagues and may not feel like there is a place for her professional voice to be heard. And yet she persists. She continuously strives to do better and be better for those around her, both personally and professionally, because she believes in her work and wants to have a positive impact on the world.

What soft small notion would you encourage other women practitioners to embrace?

I would encourage other women practitioners to find ways of disrupting the narrative that they are soft and small. I would encourage Solution Focused practitioners to find their voice and speak with pride and confidence both within and outside of their Solution Focused practice.

My best hopes for other female Solution Focused voices

My biggest aspiration for other women practising the Solution Focused approach is that they continue to find their voice and speak out. According to Morgenroth et al. (2021), leadership is an area where women continue to be underrepresented. The Solution Focused field is populated primarily by women and I hope that in the future we continue to elevate the voices of female practitioners in public forums and spaces. I hope that we as Solution Focused practitioners continue to choose differently, over and over again, and create a community of support rather than competition. Solution Focused practice is founded in mutual respect and understanding. I hope that within this network, no one voice seeks to outshine the others.

Co-constructive editors' reflections

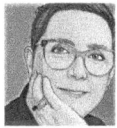 You know, I've been very interested in single sessions and I think it is interesting to have this perspective in the book. It brings in something new. Aleysa says she fell in love with hope, optimism, and respect. And I mean, who wouldn't do that? I can easily understand that when she met the Solution Focused approach she fell in love with it. She also mentions this balance between work life and family life, and her role as a mother.

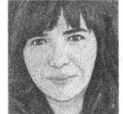 Yes, and she brings this passion for mothers and the struggles they go through into the chapter. Alesya so aptly describes how we often do not consider how difficult it is for a mother to do what we think is ordinary. And this reminds me of Insoo Kim Berg in "Hot tips" talking about how the ordinary is actually extraordinary. For some women,

the mere act of getting to therapy is an extraordinary feat and Aleysa's starting point is looking at the resilience of how people manage to come for that one session.

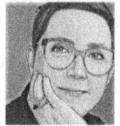

Yes, this made me think about the structures and models that are set up in organisations and departments, and how they are not always very useful. She brings in a meta-perspective on how certain structures and models are set up to help a person, but in fact are not actually helping. I am thinking of the Danish welfare system trying to be helpful and supportive, but it is a paradox. Alesya invites us to reflect on whether we are really helpful and supportive and I really, really love this.

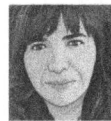

I loved that she writes that she is more interested not in what is happening, but in how people are getting to the sessions. She is already using a resource and making that hopeful resource of wanting help the centre of the conversation because she's into short, useful, hopeful, and helpful conversations.

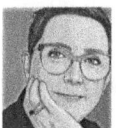

It fascinated me that she said, "For the first time in my career, I was seeing clients who were experiencing problems, both big and small, in real time". I was thinking, "Ok, when is it not real time, and what is real time?" But to pay attention to, right here and now, really pay attention, that is real time and this kind of attention, I think, is so unique in single sessions.

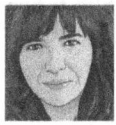

And therefore, in real time you make everything you say count, acting as if it is the first and the last session. What also really stood out for me is when Alesya writes that the Solution Focused Single Session alleviates significant amounts of stress because she is using exactly what she gets in the moment, in real time. And hope is immediate, I love that. It reminds me of Insoo Kim Berg in the Yalom interview saying she works with the hopeful side of people (Yalom & Rubin, n.d.).

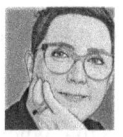

I think it's a good point, to remember that it can be stressful to have several sessions.

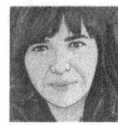

And it reminds me of what Ben Furman and Zatloukal (2022) say, when they remind us that human suffering is not necessarily a medical condition, and you do not need to come week after week. Aleysa is implying that even though the client is going through hard stuff right now, we are going to hope right now. And Aleysa has a bigger systemic look, she is aware of micro and macro levels. She looks at what is good for the client and what is good for the system, what is not good for the client and what is not good for the system.

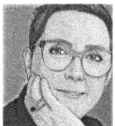

Yes, she reminds us of bridge building between systems and that we can affect not only individuals but larger communities as well. We have the ability to bring about change at both micro and macro levels. And then I was surprised that other people would notice her Solution Focused **being** in her parenting. This reminds me about a research project about Solution Focused practitioners who were also parents and how **being** Solution Focused influenced or affected their children (Kuhn, 2017), and how these values of hope and optimism transferred to their children.

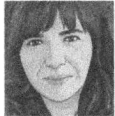

And how she brings hope, optimism, and then some kind of resilience to her children. She uses a very beautiful word; she says that, "I've transferred" it to my children so that they can see challenges as possibilities.

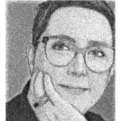

And then I really like how she differentiates between the macro and the micro levels and how Solution Focused Single Session Therapy can influence both. On a macro level it can influence social justice, and on a micro level it can create change for an individual. Also on the micro level, she is introducing us to this idea of hope or Hope Therapy, which I haven't heard about before. I mean, it was just nice to have it put this way.

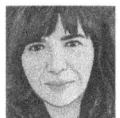

So, Solution Focused work is really ethical because it contributes to the client's own life, own goals, own ideas of treatment, and healing. And it is flexible and not imposing Western ideas on clients; thus it's a treatment in itself on that bigger macro level. If you look at Snyder's Hope Theory and how he says hope happens, then our Solution Focused questions are by default hopeful. We are thus by default **doing** hope. We are inviting hope in, doing hope, and we are helping create that flexibility that makes hope part of the process. There is thus no such thing as false hope (Snyder, 2002).

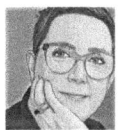

Exactly. Here in Denmark, we say it fits like a sock in a shoe; it is a match. Our questions, our way of working, our beliefs are parallel tracks to doing hope and it makes good sense. I think we are already doing it.

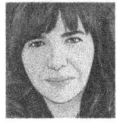

What really stood out for me, and really made me think, is that she's saying therapy and change happen outside the session and the aim of Single Session Therapy is to grow desire. It is about growing a desire for the best hope and helping the client believe that they can get there. And the more you build on and grow the level of desire for change, the more you expand on it, the more it will happen in real time.

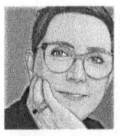 What surprised me is who inspires her. Initially I was thinking, oh, maybe we did not ask the question clearly, but then I realised it's not that she does not understand our question, it is about not highlighting anybody and acknowledging the women we haven't heard about yet.

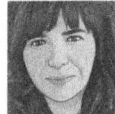 Yes, and I kind of got the idea she wrote it for the person reading it. You might be the Solution Focused practitioner – that's why you bought this book. And you might be quietly going about being undervalued. And Aleysa is saying, "You are the one who I value, who inspires me. You're the one who is continuously striving to read more, better yourself, and be a better professional. You're not seeking the spotlight, you're buying this book, reading more about it, trying to better yourself, and you're the one who inspires me."

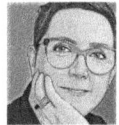 And that's a nice thought, you know, it is. It is like giving life to the book, like it can go on forever and ever. She is saying no one is better than anybody else and it complements her small notion of encouraging women to find ways of disrupting the narrative. Women are not nobody, we are not soft and small, we have a voice and we speak with pride and confidence and we are big and noisy. I really, really love that she invites us to stop talking about being soft and small.

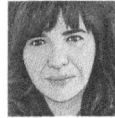 Yes, I love it too. She is encouraging us to disrupt that narrative, to find our voice, speak with pride, and create a community of support rather than competition. No one voice seeks to outshine the other; we all have value.

Author references

Cait, C.A., Skop, M., Booton, J., Stalker, C.A., Horton, S., & Riemer, M. (2017). Practice-based qualitative research: Participant experiences of walk-in counselling and traditional counselling. *Qualitative Social Work: Research and Practice*, *16*(5), 612–630.

Morgenroth, T., Ryan, M.K., Rink, F., & Begeny, C. (2021). The (in)compatibility of identities: Understanding gender differences in work–life conflict through the fit with leaders. *British Journal of Social Psychology*, *60*(2), 448–469.

Slive, A., & Bobele, M. (2011). Walking in: An aspect of everyday living. In A. Slive & M. Bobele (Eds.), *When one hour is all you have: Effective therapy for walk-in clients*(pp. 11–22). Zeig, Tucker & Theisen.

Slive, A., & Bobele, M. (2012). Walk-in counselling services: Making the most of one hour. *Australian and New Zealand Journal of Family Therapy*, *33*(01), 27–38.

Snyder, C.R. (2002). Hope Theory: Rainbows in the mind. *Psychological Inquiry*, *13*(4), 249–275.

Editor references

Berg, I.K. (n.d.). *Hot tips*. South Dakota State University. https://www.sdstate.edu/sites/defa ult/files/2018-06/hot_tips.pdf

Kuhn, K. (2017). *Exploring educational psychologists' personal relationships in their families using Solution Focused therapy*. [M.Ed Psych. thesis, University of Johannesburg] https://ujcontent.uj.ac.za/view/pdfCoverPage?instCode=27UOJ_INST&filePid=1361 56260007691&download=true

Mo, Y.L. (2013, 3 September). Solution Focused Brief Therapy. In *Encyclopaedia of Social Work*. https://doi.org/10.1093/acrefore/9780199975839.013.1039

Yalom, V., & Rubin, B. (n.d.). *Insoo Kim Berg on Solution Focused Brief Therapy*. Psychotherapy.Net. https://www.psychotherapy.net/interview/insoo-kim-berg

Zatloukal, L., & Furman, B. (2022). The Solution-Focused approach to trauma therapy. *Journal of Constructivist Psychology*. https://doi.org/10.1080/10720537.2022.2035863

Chapter 7

A way to unlock potential and strengthen cooperation

A Solution Focused perspective in a school context in Germany

Katrin Berger (Germany)

Introduction

For me, the Solution Focused approach was love at first sight and allowed me to rediscover ways of being that I intuitively chose as a child. This has allowed me to follow my own bodily resonance and not the expectations of others. I have learnt to give my attention and energy to what feels right and alive, which makes my work deeply meaningful. I support and collaborate with schools using the Solution Focused method of Berg and Shilts (2005) called the WOWW (Working on What Works) Class Coaching model.

Reflect on how your gender influences your work–life and being a Solution Focused practitioner

I grew up in a rural area with two brothers and many other children around me. This allowed me to try out different activities, some more associated with boys and others that were considered typically female. I didn't think about it, but followed my desire to learn. I see that as a great gift. The adults in my life, who were inevitably also my role models, showed something very different, however, in their activities and the distribution of their tasks. The women in my life were either busy with household and family work or with professional childcare. This made them financially dependent on the main breadwinner and limited their personal room for growth and learning – and possibly also love. Consequently, financial independence is something to which I aspire and I am always looking for people who exemplify equality in their everyday lives and relationships in a very practical way.

After my studies in adult education, I worked as a municipal equality officer while raising my eight-year-old son as a single parent. I was concerned about inequality and tried to work effectively for more equality. In the process, I realised that many things are so structurally ingrained that it is not enough to look at the individual and appeal for change. It also needs good networks and legislation and, in the best-case scenario, Solution Focused methods and processes. Luckily, I already had some Solution Focused training, and at a local political event I asked the miracle question: "Suppose equal rights for women and men became a reality

DOI: 10.4324/9781003430254-8

overnight – how would we notice it in concrete terms?" Everyone experienced this as a new way to exchange ideas and I learned an incredible amount in this job, especially how important good cooperation and networks are and how much can be achieved with a small budget, good ideas, committed complementary companions, and strong motivation. I was also able to build on this learning experience in later career roles.

As I mentioned, the Solution Focused approach was love at first sight for me and allowed me to rediscover the Solution Focused methods I had used as a child. As a child, I framed unattractive but unavoidable tasks, such as cleaning the bathroom, in such a way that they became interesting and pleasurable games. I collected positive experiences and observations in a diary and, together with friends, founded a support group for neighbourhood animals. Perhaps this is also the reason why I enjoy working with children so much today, as children often act very intuitively towards their own solutions.

In all my subsequent activities, as a family therapist and mediator, working with families, as a team leader in the field of youth welfare (child protection), and even in my current role working with schools, the focus on solutions has run through my work like a red thread.

I find it difficult to say what this has to do with my gender. I don't like to assign characteristics and behaviours to a certain gender, in order not to reinforce restrictive attributions. However, what has become very clear to me in answering this question is that women, at least here in Germany, are still disadvantaged (in terms of salaries, pensions, leadership positions, share of family work, and public visibility). In this respect, as a woman and as a Solution Focused practitioner, I am committed to supporting fairness where disadvantage is experienced and to increasing self-responsibility and self-efficacy.

I cannot say whether I work differently than men, but I am aware that emotional care is important to me personally and that I feel more connected to Insoo Kim Berg than to the sobriety of Steve de Shazer. I have also noticed that I am strongly motivated when I experience something as meaningful for a better world and that I generously share knowledge and materials, just as others have shared with me. The thrill I get from eye-to-eye cooperation is greater than the thrill I get from highlighting myself and my importance. I wish that this were neither feminine nor masculine, but simply human.

What is your good reason for staying a Solution Focused practitioner?

I identify as a Solution Focused practitioner, yet, at the same time, I don't actually call myself that. When I witnessed arguments among Solution Focused practitioners many years ago about what was Solution Focused and what was not, it unsettled me. What is the unifying factor? How do we define it? Who decides?

Certainly, a discussion about what it is and what it is not can give direction to the approach and contribute to the term "Solution Focused" not becoming arbitrary.

However, a definition can also be restrictive and promote rigid standardisation. Since I admire diversity and shy away from constriction, I have not concerned myself too much with whether I am doing it right and have mainly given myself over to my desire to learn in practice. At the same time, I feel I belong to the imaginary "international association of Solution Focused practitioners".

And indeed, the desire to learn is the main reason why I keep the red Solution Focused thread in my work. For me, a Solution Focused framing of an interactive exchange is the ground on which learning can take place without fear and rather with trust and the joy of experimenting. This is how I experienced it in my Solution Focused training, and this is how I would like to convey it in my work. Even in my private life the red thread shines through and brings lightness into my relationships. In my understanding, Solution Focused work is a kind of well-meaning liquefaction process. As we explore, shape, and consolidate a desired interaction with each other, what no longer fits casually liquefies. A new form is created that is fit for the moment.

What would others notice you doing that would tell them that you work from a Solution Focused approach?

When I am working with children or adults in a counselling situation, I ask about their desired future. I support them in seeing their own situation as a hopeful, positive, and resource-rich base. Often there is already so much success that we can build upon.

Children and young people experience me as encouraging, positive, and optimistic, whether that is as an observer of what works in the school lesson, or during the break, or gathering their feedback at the end of the lesson as part of WOWW Class Coaching (Berg & Shilts, 2005). I offer a structure that makes good intentions and skills visible. I try to empower young people and teachers towards an appreciative interaction, to enable them to implement WOWW on their own and soon make myself redundant.

I can also be seen putting in place a support group for an unhappy primary school child, either using Sue Young's (2011) approach to stop bullying or the Kids' Skills training by Ben Furman (2016). In both cases, I am concerned with reinforcing or initiating an interaction of success, as well as expanding the individual's range of action and experiencing choices.

In case conferences, when people are contributing their different views of a situation, I am particularly interested in noticing what has already succeeded and in exceptions to the problem, or the possible good reasons for the current problematic behaviour. In addition, I invite all participants to look at what connects them, their hopes, abilities, and goals. I often ask, "How will we know specifically that the situation is good enough?" I make sure that everyone's contributions are named and reinforced as valuable. In all the contexts mentioned, I use the Solution Focused scale (1–10, goal achievement or confidence). This allows different perspectives to be presented in a condensed way to start with and to be expanded going forward.

Since this type of case conference has already been experienced as helpful, I am often given the task of moderating. This enables even more Solution Focused framing than when I am merely a participant.

Share an exercise that might be useful to other women practitioners

WOWW Class Coaching

I have taken up the basic idea of WOWW and adapted it to my work context by developing a structured process that actively involves the children and young people as observers of what works from the very beginning. My driving idea was to make it possible to experience the Solution Focused approach as directly as possible and to motivate the participants to invent their own methods and frameworks with the focus they have learned. I would like to achieve sustainability in relation to Solution Focusing, which is apparent in independent implementation as well as in the adaptation to the respective context. I usually support a class for about half a year, one lesson per week.

- In the first phase, I am guided by the teacher's goal. The class learns to look at the desired behaviour and to give each other encouraging feedback.
- In the second phase, the children and young people develop an idea of their community at its best and decide on their own class goal in a workshop. They then mainly observe the desired behaviour that fits their own goal, and increasingly take the lead in their own WOWW lessons.
- In the third phase, I observe them doing it on their own. I find even children and young people can take over the WOWW programme. I can then hand out a WOWW certificate to the class and say goodbye.

WOWW is suitable for both primary and secondary schools. Currently, I am also experimenting with having the process carried out entirely without external observers.

Share how you adapt the approach and make it your own. Give us five characteristics that are a part of your Solution Focused DNA

I learned the Solution Focused approach in a setting oriented towards the Solution Focused Brief Therapy approach from Milwaukee. I also studied the hypnosystemic approach by Gunter Schmidt, as well as conflict resolution and mediation, including the relationship-oriented approach of Thomas Gordon. I have also added the playfulness of improvisational theatre. These other approaches have been added to a greater or lesser extent to create a wonderful fusion.

The five central aspects of my personal Solution Focused DNA:

Humour: in almost everything I do as a Solution Focused practitioner, I enjoy contributing to laughing together. I find it builds relationships when one risks showing a sense of humour with another. And if things go wrong, I can at least laugh at myself and thus take away some of the horror of failure in our relationships and learning space.

Incorporating sensory experiences: I like to take my existing Solution Focused methods in a direction where even more senses are activated. For the WOWW process, I use posters that the children often create themselves. I use colourful balls that make the feedback more fun, and I incorporate interaction games, team games, music, and improvisational theatre when setting goals.

A broader focus: there was a time when I looked more enthusiastically and confidently at my clients with Solution Focused questions than they could (sustain) themselves. This led, for example, to highly contentious parents who were in the process of separating, joining me in my enthusiasm for mediation and once even kissing afterwards in the car park of the counselling centre. At the next appointment they came back even more divided. I have learned from this. Today, I look more calmly and serenely at the resources and goals of the other person while also seeing the contradictions and ambivalences. This can sometimes seem a little problem-focused; however, I call it looking lovingly with a larger picture. In the end, I find myself being of more help to clients.

Ask questions, listen, and build on each other: perhaps because I love good stories and fundamentally like people, I got into the habit early on of asking questions with which I can elicit stories. In this way, I can contribute to making a conversation enriching. Experiencing how the storytellers then talk with shining eyes about things that are important to them spurs me on to stick with it.

In a private context, it also makes me particularly happy when my stories are teased out and shared in a conversation and both sides relate to each other and the trains of thought build on each other. This is not specifically Solution Focused for now, but it is 100% part of my personal DNA as a Solution Focused practitioner.

Encouraging interaction: in my work, I experience how the community can be strengthened and the learning potential increased when all the children in a class have learned to work in different groups with all their classmates. By encouraging interaction, I am constantly learning and teaching at the same time. I am always driven by the question, "How can we increase interaction and independence while maintaining the joy of learning together as a class in the longer term?"

Which female practitioner inspires you and in which way?

Many female practitioners inspire me, such as the two editors of this empowering book project, which also encourages networking. However, three women in particular have inspired and influenced me:

Firstly, Insoo Kim Berg. Reading her books and watching her videos have given an extra bit of heart, compassion, and vitality to the Solution Focused structure.

Secondly, Sue Young, from the United Kingdom. After three years of Solution Focused training, I met Sue and her Solution Focused approach to addressing bullying in schools. Watching how Sue works with children in a peer-support group, I could immediately see how finely she observes, how much she loves children, and how she trusts their creativity and willingness to help. Sue considers so many things that I think are very important for the effectiveness and sustainability of the method, for example, the ongoing involvement of parents and teachers. She strongly promotes the creation of a friendly, interactive class and school culture which, after occasional support from the group, can then stabilise the well-being of the child concerned in the longer term and benefit everyone involved.

I have had the opportunity to work with her on aligning a school team in a Solution Focused way and this collaboration has developed into a friendly relationship that continues to this day. I have been able to support her in work projects and assignments and she has supported me in different ways. When Sue was unable to carry out assignments, she felt confident to pass them on to me. To feel that I am trusted, perhaps even a little more than I trust myself, is very inviting for growth and for a relationship that is characterised by appreciation, gratitude, and the desire to give back or pass on.

Thirdly, Katalin Hankovszky – she is a source of inspiration. Katalin has been running training courses in Solution Focused Learning Coaching for teachers in Bremen for many years. When we discovered that we both work with Bremen's schools, we decided to start a regional network called Solution Focus in Schools in Bremen. Since 2020 this network has served to encourage Solution Focused professionals working in the school context. In addition, Katalin and I occasionally involve each other in work assignments, which I find very enriching. I am always inspired by the way she continuously brings people into new constellations of conversations with Solution Focused questions and intuitive ease. Katalin is committed to focusing on what is already happening in the here and now in terms of desired change. She seems to be consistently searching for the essence of the Solution Focus and is thus a very exciting colleague in the learning process.

I am very grateful to these three women and to all the other people who network in a Solution Focused way and generously give their knowledge and trust.

What soft small notion would you encourage other women practitioners to embrace?

It has become increasingly important for me to see what my own bodily resonance is when I do something. I want to be less worried over rules of politeness or the possible expectations of others. Where I feel alive, where I experience the doing as pleasurable and easy, or where it is deeply meaningful to me – that's where I give my attention and energy. This is not out of egoism, but because I am convinced that is when we achieve the most. I would like to encourage other women to do the same.

Share your best hopes for other female Solution Focused voices

Als ich kürzlich mit Katalin über diese Frage sprach, war meine Antwort eine große, ambitionierte Hoffnung. Ich dachte im Sinne der von mir gestellten Wunderfrage im politischen Kontext, an die großen globalen Herausforderungen. Wie könnten diese mit lösungsfokussierten Prozessen in eine Richtung gestaltet werden, die möglichst vielen Menschen und zukünftigen Generationen ein gutes Leben ermöglicht? Frauen könnten hier eine besondere Rolle spielen, weil sie möglicherweise mehr sinnorientiert und sozial abgestimmt zu handeln gelernt haben. Meine Hoffnung ist, dass Frauen sich in ihren Arbeits- und Lebensbereichen, in denen sie sich lebendig und sinnerfüllt erleben, aktiv vernetzen, sichtbar und öffentlich werden, großzügig ihr Wissen teilen und zugleich auch sich selbstverantwortlich um die eigene Lernlust kümmern.

Und als ich dann neugierig fragte, was Katalins Antwort wäre, sagte sie: "Dass Frauen Freude haben mit dem, was sie tun!". Da musste ich innerlich lachen. Der ganz große Entwurf oder die ganz kleinen Schritte. Vielleicht brauchen wir ja beides!

When I recently spoke to Katalin about this question, my answer was one of great, ambitious hope. I was thinking in terms of the "miracle question" in the political context of major global challenges. How could these challenges be shaped with Solution Focused processes in a direction that enables as many people and future generations as possible to live well? Women could play a special role here because they may have learned to act in a more meaning-oriented and socially coordinated way. My hope is that women will actively network, become visible and public in their fields of work and life where they feel alive and meaningful, generously share their knowledge, and, at the same time, take responsibility for their own desire to learn.

And when I then asked out of curiosity what Katalin's answer would be, she said: "That women have joy in what they do!" I had to laugh inside. The very grand design or the very small steps. Maybe we need both!

Co-constructive editors' reflection

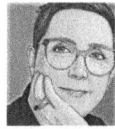 It was interesting to read that Katrin also answers the first question by going back in time and talking about her childhood. I think there is a process in answering this question; it is as though you need to step back and then step back again and back in time and reflect upon your gender when you were a child and add small layers to where you are today.

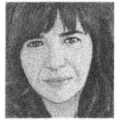 Yes, putting it in the context of time, just like we said in Chapter 1, that our Solution Focused DNA is also found in our context and time.

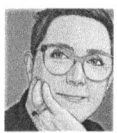 I loved that she said that she had already developed her own Solution Focused methods as a child. What a clever child, what a brilliant child! Oh, wow. She made all tasks a pleasurable game.

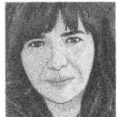

I loved that she was already doing it as a child. I also wrote that she was pretending to belong to an international association of Solution Focused people. I love that she does it in her own way, keeping the Solution Focused assumptions as her red thread. Using her own imagination and the imagination of the child reminds me of Elke Gybels (2021, p. 148) saying, "Imagination is one of the most powerful tools of the human mind".

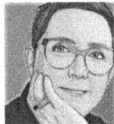

Katrin piqued my curiosity when she asked how we define the Solution Focused approach, and thus what a purist Solution Focused therapist looks like. We have discussed this several times in EBTA, and set up a task group, Theory of Practice, which has worked to find common factors, such as co-constructing with the client, having a not-knowing stance, etc. This led to the publication of a book in 2020; however, many are cautious about answering the question. It is as though that question can only be answered by Steve de Shazer.

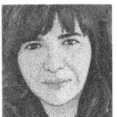

Yet, she mentions Insoo Kim Berg giving her an extra bit of heart and compassion and I love that she acknowledges Insoo in her chapter. And I also love that she says she is Solution **Focusing.** She has turned the attention into a verb – something she is constantly doing, she's constantly searching for what is working and what has already worked – Yasmin Ajmal's (2021, p. 36) looking for "pertinent sparkles". And if you do that everything else falls away and becomes irrelevant, which reminds me of Linda Metcalf (2021, p. 73) saying that finding those exceptions "reminds the teacher and student to summarise and notice times when school went better".

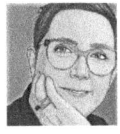

She insists that it is an active action. Her DNA is an active focus. And I love being reminded to be creative, especially when working with children and in the school context. She has so many different tools in her toolbox that she adapts to any kind of situation with the child, while always being Solution Focused.

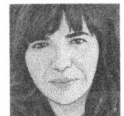

Yes, and what really stood out for me is Katrin uses humour and other sensory experiences, which reminds me of Tina Rae et al. (2018, p. 19) saying that using all the senses "conveys an understanding that is more powerful than words". She really focuses on the interaction between two people. For Katrin, Solution Focusing is a desired interaction, this co-constructing between people; it's almost as though she is saying that we need to be mindful of how people interact and our goal needs to be to help people to interact differently.

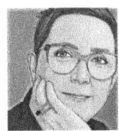

Katrin has made the approach her own and I love it when she says, "Look lovingly at the bigger picture", almost as though she is saying that if she looks with a wider lens then she can do Solution Focusing because she doesn't ignore problems.

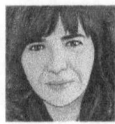 And then I love how she ends the chapter with a journey of inspiration. She starts with Insoo Kim Berg and then mentions other women who are still influencing her today, as though she is taking us on this journey with her.

Author references

Berg, I.K., & Shilts, L. (2005). *The WOWW approach: Handbook for Solution-Focused teaching strategies (simple but not easy)*. Brief Family Therapy Center.

Furman, B. (2016). *Kids' Skills: Playful and practical solution-finding with children*. St Luke's Innovative Resources.

Young, S. (2011). *Solution-Focused schools: Anti-bullying and beyond*. BT Press.

Editor references

Ajmal, Y. (2021). From challenging to outstanding. In D. Yusuf (Ed.), *The Solution Focused approach with children and young people*. Routledge.

Gybels, E., & Prenen, R. (2021). Figuring future: The art of reframing challenges. In D. Yusuf (Ed.), *The Solution Focused approach with children and young people*. Routledge.

Metcalf, L. (2021). A Solution Focused team conversation. In D. Yusuf (Ed.), *The Solution Focused approach with children and young people*. Routledge.

Rae, T., Thomas, M., & Walshe, J. (2018). *The essential guide to using Solution Focused Brief Therapy with children and adolescents*. Hinton House.

Sundman, P., Schwab, M., Wolf, F., Wheeler, J., Cabié, M.-C., van der Hoorn, S., Pakrosnis, R., Dierolf, K., & Hjerth, M. (2020). *Theory of Solution-Focused practice: Version 2020*. European Brief Therapy Association.

Chapter 8

Keep it simple

A few words about Solution Focused therapy

Marie-Carmen Neipp (Spain)

Introduction

I lecture in the Department of Health Psychology at the Miguel Hernández University of Elche in Spain. My field of interest is health psychology, focusing on the study of psychosocial variables such as beliefs, coping, social support, and communication, as well as their influence on people's quality of life and well-being. My aim is to empower people to manage their problematic situations successfully, and the relative simplicity of the approach helps me do so. In recent years I have focused my research on the application of Solution Focused therapy and Positive Psychology techniques in different fields.

Reflect on how your gender influences your work–life and being a Solution Focused practitioner

Being a woman allows me to establish emotional connections with clients. Women are generally more aware of their emotions, which can help me connect better with clients' feelings, creating a more open and receptive therapeutic environment. Additionally, being a woman also helps me establish a trusting relationship with clients or colleagues more easily.

Furthermore, being a woman influences how I view and construct the world around me, attempting to be more resilient, empathetic, and understanding of people's unique experiences. Therefore, I emphasise using empowering language to help clients discover their resources and strengths so they can use them to cope with their problems and improve their emotional well-being and quality of life.

What is your good reason for staying a Solution Focused practitioner?

I have always been a positive and optimistic person who focuses on living in the present. When I started my psychology training, none of the therapeutic perspectives taught resonated with me until I discovered the Solution Focused Brief Therapy approach in the final year of my degree.

DOI: 10.4324/9781003430254-9

In 2012, I began an intensive training programme in Solution Focused Brief Therapy directed by Dr Mark Beyebach and Dr Marga Herrero de Vega. As a result, I acquired more knowledge, techniques, and resources and obtained the title of Advanced Solution-Focused Practitioner. Since then, I have been combining my academic work with clinical practice.

My research at the university focuses on studying psychosocial variables (beliefs, coping, social support, communication, etc.) and their influence on individuals' well-being, mainly in the health field. With my training in Solution Focused Brief Therapy, I thought it would be interesting to apply some of its techniques in the health context. I contacted my former professor and now friend, Dr Mark Beyebach, proposing a collaboration. Since 2014, we have carried out various reviews of and research on Solution Focused Brief Therapy.

We have adapted and validated the Solution Focused inventory, which evaluates different Solution Focused thoughts (Neipp et al., 2017), and analysed the differential impact of various types of Solution Focused Brief Therapy questions (miracle, exception, and scaling) compared to problem-focused questions (Neipp et al., 2016; Neipp et al., 2021). We have also trained nurses in Solution Focused communication, showing that this type of communication significantly influenced the increase in fluid adherence in haemodialysis patients (Beyebach et al., 2018). Finally, we conducted a bibliometric analysis (Beyebach et al., 2021) and a literature review of Solution Focused Brief Therapy (Neipp & Beyebach, 2022). The results confirm the worldwide applicability and efficacy of Solution Focused Brief Therapy as a single or main component of psychosocial interventions.

In conclusion, based on my experience in clinical practice and research, I consider that I continue to apply, teach, and research Solution Focused Brief Therapy mainly for personal reasons and my clinical practice, focusing on people's resources and strengths to help them seek solutions and solve their problems. It is also a way to empower people to proactively manage their problematic situations successfully. In addition, and related to training and research, thanks to the relative simplicity of the different Solution Focused questions we can train a broad variety of professionals from different fields (healthcare, education, organisations, etc.) to include this type of questioning in their professional practice and help people better adapt to their situations.

What would others notice you doing that would tell them that you work from a Solution Focused approach?

I think they notice it mainly by how I handle difficulties that arise at work. I try to redefine the situation, transforming it from a difficulty into an opportunity to learn and grow. I focus on searching for possible solutions, selecting the simplest one to implement, and trying to overcome the difficulty.

In addition, when I work on a team, I try to identify the small contributions each team member makes to the work to highlight and publicly recognise them. This way, I try to ensure that everyone is aware that they have contributed something, no matter how little, and that they feel valued in their work.

I also believe that they perceive that I work from a Solution Focused approach by how I use language, knowing that the language used to talk about a problem differs from the language used to talk about solutions. I tend to focus more on asking how people do things rather than why they do them.

Share an exercise that might be useful to other women practitioners

This task comes from the book *200 tasks in Brief Therapy* by Beyebach and Herrero de la Vega (2010), two outstanding Spanish Solution Focused therapists.

The letter from the future

Task description: the client is encouraged to write a letter to herself from the future, 20 or 30 years ahead, thinking she has overcome the problems that brought her to therapy, and is an older and wiser version of herself. In this letter, she encourages her current self and tells her how she managed to get through it, who helped her, and what personal qualities she could use.

This exercise could be useful for hopeless clients focused on their distressing present. The goal is to broaden their time perspective and generate expectations of success. In addition, the advice given to herself from the future can help create interesting alternatives in the present. This task can be used in any stage of change and at almost any time in therapy. The book's authors learned this task from Yvonne Dolan (Dolan, 1991), who, in turn, collected it from Capachione (1979). An interesting variant is to use this task at the end of therapy as a resource to prevent relapse. It is called "the congratulation letter". This letter is written from the near future, six months or one year later. In the letter, the person congratulates herself for continuing to do the things she knows help her, and describes them in detail. When the established time frame (six months, one year) is up, the client rereads the letter. Thus it could function as a "self-session".

Share how you adapt the approach and make it your own. Give us five characteristics that are a part of your Solution Focused DNA

Working with emotions: while training as a Solution Focused therapist, I read Eve Lipchik's book *Beyond technique in Solution-Focused therapy: Working with emotions and the therapeutic relationship* (2002). From then on, I embraced many of Lipchik's proposals for working with emotions in therapy. Eve suggested that therapists should explicitly talk to clients about feelings, as they are inseparable from behaviour and cognition. In this sense, throughout the therapy session, I am interested not only in observable behaviours but also in the emotional aspects of the process, as emotions can facilitate solutions by providing an important means of connecting with and understanding clients.

Interactive process: following Eve's proposal, I consider my conversations with clients as an interactive process. In this process, the problem and possible solutions gradually interweave into a plot that will ultimately represent the solution for the client. Therefore, based on my experience, when clients find it difficult to stop talking about problems, talking about their feelings can create an emotional climate suitable for redefining the problematic situation and bridging the gap to start discussing possible solutions.

Metaphors: these are a handy tool in helping people understand the process they are going through. Using metaphors congruent with their lifestyle, characteristics, and qualities can help people better understand the message I want to convey so they can assume control of their change process and actively engage in it. It is also useful for clients to make different associations and generate new solutions.

Intentional use of language: as a Solution Focused therapist, I believe that language is the main tool we work with in therapy. The intentional use of language aims to achieve what I propose in each therapy phase more effectively. I use clients' language, often employing expressions and terms that the client uses during the conversation to create a good therapeutic alliance. Additionally, I use expressions that are consistent with their way of constructing reality. I also try to channel clients' language, starting from their descriptions, to gradually transform their narratives and obtain new descriptions in small, concrete, interactional, and positive terms.

Symptom prescriptions or paradoxical tasks: sometimes, depending on the client's situation and characteristics, I use techniques derived from other therapeutic approaches. For example, if clients are not improving because they are trapped in a vicious circle in which the more effort they put into solving their problems the bigger they become – that is, attempted solutions become the problem – I often use "symptom prescriptions" or "paradoxical tasks", following the authors of the MRI of Palo Alto (Fisch et al., 1982). Another technique I use is "externalisation", which comes from the narrative therapeutic approach (White & Epston, 1990). It is useful when a person has a problem that paralyses them, and they cannot see beyond it. During the externalisation process, a space is created between the problem and the person, such that the problem becomes its own entity. Then the person can assume an active role and confront the problem, changing how they perceive it and their relationship with it.

Which female practitioner inspires you and in which way?

The woman who has inspired me the most in my work as a therapist is Insoo Kim Berg. I learned a lot from her by reading her books and watching various videos of her conducting therapy (Andrewstrainingvideo, 2011). I really liked her calm and slow-paced style throughout the interview and how she conveyed that calmness and built a therapeutic alliance to create a suitable environment for the session to develop. I also liked how she redirected conversations to focus more on solutions. And, last but not least, I learned from her genuine and creative way of designing and suggesting tasks for the clients.

What soft small notion would you encourage other women practitioners to embrace?

I consider language to be our main tool, so I would suggest that they pay attention to the language they use, always trying to use empowering language, and conveying to clients the message that change is inevitable because they are seeking therapy and they are on the right path to solve their problems.

Furthermore, I would include the use of compliments. I think it is important in any phase of the session to emphasise clients' positive aspects, mainly what they are already doing well to solve the problem, and also their behaviours and ideas that emerge during the session. This technique pursues several objectives: a) promoting personal competence by reinforcing the idea that individuals have the necessary resources and skills to manage and resolve their problematic situations; b) generating optimism and hope; and c) helping to improve the therapeutic relationship (Beyebach, 2014).

My best hopes for other female Solution Focused voices

Las mujeres que trabajan desde el enfoque centrado en soluciones, son un ejemplo inspirador de valentía, determinación y compromiso para la creación de un futuro mejor para todas las personas. Centrarse en las soluciones, en lugar de en los problemas, es un recordatorio constante de que cada desafío presenta una oportunidad única para innovar, colaborar y crecer tanto a nivel personal como profesional. El trabajo que las mujeres centradas en soluciones realizan es valorado y apreciado por todas las personas a las que han ayudado y siguen ayudando inspirando así, a otras mujeres a formarse y trabajar desde este enfoque.

Women working from a Solution Focused approach are an inspiring example of courage, determination, and commitment to creating a better future for all people. Focusing on solutions, rather than problems, is a constant reminder that every challenge presents a unique opportunity to innovate, collaborate, and grow, both personally and professionally. The work that Solution Focused women do is valued and appreciated by all the people they have helped and continue to help, inspiring other women to learn and work from this approach.

Co-constructive editors' reflection

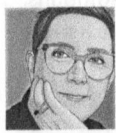

I would just love to spend more time with Marie-Carmen – her chapter is so simple and straightforward, so hands-on. She truly stands by the belief that being a woman makes a difference.

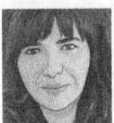

I agree with you – it's pragmatic, not fluffy, and yet brilliant. And that being a woman makes her open to emotions, and for her that openness creates what she calls a *receptive therapeutic environment.*

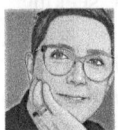

That is so nicely put, and this stance influences her beliefs and views, how she constructs. I like the word constructing; it's so vivid, fluid, changeable, and yet an active verb; we construct.

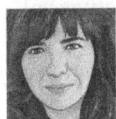

Marie-Carmen always comes from a place of present; she starts with the here and now. I absolutely loved when she wrote, "It is an approach that *proactively helps empower the client to manage problems*". And I remember when Elliott Connie, Adam Froerer, Johnny Kim, and I wrote the book about trauma, we really struggled with the title and we came up with *SFBT and clients managing trauma*, that word *manage*, not clients who have been through trauma, not clients who have experienced trauma, but clients who have managed trauma. It boils down to that presupposition, that people manage their lives.

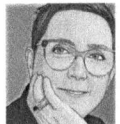

I underlined the same sentence. To *proactively manage their problematic situation successfully.* Oh, wow, I was so fascinated by that sentence. I was surprised because I realised something, maybe for the first time: this is not only about moving forward but also about managing and coping with a problematic situation. I see it all the time, that there is a tendency to make the Solution Focused approach more about action planning: what would it take to move from four to five? What would a first step be? In a way pushing the client. *Managing* just allows us to be in the present with the client, right here and now, and not just moving forward.

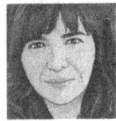

Yes, and I think she tells us exactly how she does that; she tells us so beautifully how she helps clients manage difficult situations. She redefines the difficulties as opportunities. She uses hope language all the time. What is fascinating about her chapter for me is that I have always taught about hope-catching language, but Marie-Carmen says she is actively teaching her clients hope language and that she is transforming their language.

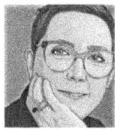 Which reminds me about the significant work on microanalysis from Janet Bavelas, among others, micro-analysing the language and the co-construction of the language; looking into which words we can preserve, enlarge, or reduce.

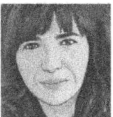 It is all about what a therapist does within a session. But Marie-Carmen is going one step further and says, yes, we can look at our own language, but we can also – and her words here are intentional – transform their words. I love that.

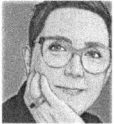 Still within the framework of microanalysis; to make invitations to the client and not only build upon their language, because research shows that Solution Focused practitioners use and build upon the client's words in a significant way. I think she is really paying attention to all the language the client uses and I can really relate to that, as all we have is the language. She is so aware of her own use of words throughout the whole chapter, such as "transforming it from difficulties into an opportunity to learn and grow". That's what it is, an example of the chapter's simplicity: there are only the words that are needed.

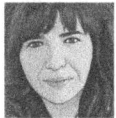 There is no fluff here. I just loved what you just said: no more words than what is needed.

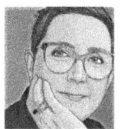 Something else reminded me of Steve de Shazer: "I tend to focus more and ask how people do things rather than why they do it". And that is one of the things I've been taught as well. Marie-Carmen reminds us that whenever you ask how people are doing something, they tend to answer with why they are doing it, and therefore we have to ask the same questions several times.

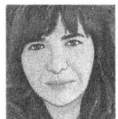 And another thing she puts into her chapter that I personally really value is her ability as a woman to work with emotions. She said she explicitly talks about emotions in her session because she believes it bridges the gap to possibility. It's an interactive process, you *interweave* the emotions into the plot. I love that. And by doing that, when you talk explicitly about emotions, then you start redefining the situation and building a bridge to possibility.

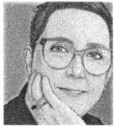 Yes, and for me this is different from the work at BRIEF and the paper by Mark McKergow on SFBT 2.0, which talks about descriptions of actions and behaviour and, in a way, turns the approach into a descriptive approach. What Marie-Carmen writes about goes a bit beyond that, as she writes about what is in between one behaviour and another

behaviour, what connects one action with another. We are back to "in between", and what links different kinds of actions are emotions. She allows herself and us to explore what is in between behaviours, which in a sense gives more value.

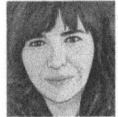

And for me that in-between space is not a linear space; rather it is a flexible weaving between emotion, behaviour, and possibility.

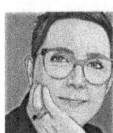

Yes, back and forth, back and forth, like when I'm knitting, backward and forward …

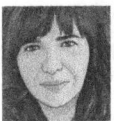

Which reminds me of stacking – you are stacking, and as you're doing it new ideas emerge. It is a constant stacking and weaving, stacking and weaving, linking the stitches together, and then a new pattern emerges, a redefinition emerges. She also integrates other things in that interweaving conversation; she might use a metaphor, she might use externalisation, or she'll go and search for anything else to continue the weaving in between.

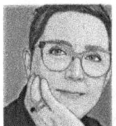

Beautifully said. When I'm knitting I use different kinds of yarns, or add some patterns, and the process is still knitting. There is still a product, a blouse, or a shawl as a result.

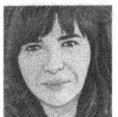

I agree – the colours you add, the yarn you add, the metaphors you add, those additions are all intentional because they are creating language that transforms. And two other things that come out for me in this chapter are hope and compliments.

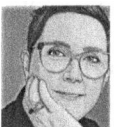

Yes, how a powerful language creates hope. That we can use language that empowers the client and brings hope – which, I think, compliments do too. Her way of working is grounded in her experiences, in her research, and in her clear ideas and convictions. And I got curious. I would like to read the research by Mark Beyebach on compliments because there are different opinions on how to use compliments, whether we should use it, when to use it, and what exactly is a compliment. Marie-Carmen's input is inspiring.

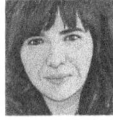

Yes, and it's also nice when you read something and think, this is a re-reminder. I need to go back to re-examine the use of compliments, the use of intentionally transforming language for the client with the client. It is nice to get an aha moment, and to discover I want to do more of it, or I want to explore this again.

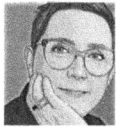 And then she says, "The work that Solution Focused women do is valued and appreciated by all the people they have helped and continue to help". Wow, this reminded me about the good reason, why we are doing what we do, that our co-constructive conversations are useful. We are writing a book for professionals with professionals, and she reminds us that we have a client and that it is all about the client. It is basically about helping other people struggling with their lives, and that is such a nice thought.

Author references

Andrewstrainingvideo. (2011, 1 April). *Solution focus: Solutions step by step* [Video]. YouTube. https://www.youtube.com/watch?v=tjdJhdA9mE4&t=38s

Beyebach, M. (2014). *24 ideas para una psicoteraia breve.* (2nd ed.). Herder.

Beyebach, M., & Herrero de la Vega, M. (2010). *200 tareas en terapia breve.* Herder.

Beyebach, M., Neipp, M.C., García, M., & González, I. (2018). Impact of nurses' Solution-Focused communication on the fluid adherence of adult patients on hemodialysis. *Journal of Advanced Nursing, 74*, 2654–2657. https://doi.org/10.1111/jan.13792

Beyebach, M., Neipp, M.C., Solanes-Puchol, A., & Martín-del-Río, B. (2021). Bibliometric differences between WEIRD and non-WEIRD countries in the outcome research on Solution-Focused Brief Therapy. *Frontiers in Psychology, 12*, 754885. https://doi.org/10.3389/fpsyg.2021.754885

Capachione, L. (1979). *The creative journal: The art of finding yourself.* Ohio University Press.

Dolan, Y. (1991). *Resolving sexual abuse.* Norton.

Fisch, R., Weakland, J.H., & Segal, L. (1982). *The tactics of change: Doing therapy briefly.* Jossey-Bass.

Kiser, D.J., Piercy, F.P., & Lipchik, E. (1993). The integration of emotions in Solution-Focused therapy. *Journal of Marital and Family Therapy, 19*(3), 233–242.

Lipchik, E. (2002). *Beyond technique in Solution-Focused therapy: Working with emotions and the therapeutic relationship.* Guilford Press.

Neipp, M.C., & Beyebach, M. (2022). The global outcomes of Solution-Focused Brief Therapy: A revision. *The American Journal of Family Therapy.* https://doi.org/10.1080/01926187.2022.2069175

Neipp, M.C., Beyebach, M., Nuñez, R., & Martínez-González, M.C. (2016). The effect of Solution-Focused versus problem-focused questions: A replication. *Journal of Marital and Family Therapy, 42*(3), 525–535. https://doi.org/10.1111/jmft.12140

Neipp, M.C., Beyebach, M., Sánchez-Prada, A., & Delgado-Álvarez, C. (2021). Solution-Focused versus problem-focused questions: Differential effects of miracles, exceptions and scales. *Journal of Family Therapy, 43*, 728–747. https://doi.org/10.1111/1467-6427.12345

Neipp, M.C., Tirado, S., Beyebach, M., & Martínez-González, M.C. (2017). Spanish adaptation of the Solution-Focused Inventory (SFI). *Terapia Psicológica, 35*(1), 5–14. https://doi.org/10.4067/S0718-48082017000100001

White, M., & Epston, D. (1990). *Narrative means to therapeutic ends.* Dulwich Centre Publications.

Editor references

De Jong, P., Bavelas, J.B., & Kormann, H. (2013). An introduction to using microanalysis to observe co-construction in psychotherapy. *Journal of Systemic Therapies*, *32*(3), s. 17–30.

Jordan, S.S., Froerer, A.S., & Bavelas, J.B. (2013). Microanalysis of positive and negative content in Solution-Focused Brief Therapy and Cognitive Behavioral Therapy expert sessions. *Journal of Systemic Therapies*, *32*(3), 46–59.

McKergow, M. (2016). SFBT 2.0: The next generation of Solution Focused Brief Therapy has already arrived. *Journal of Solution Focused Brief Therapy*, *2*(2), 1–17.

Chapter 9

It's a kind of magic

Solution Focused practice with children and families

Ursula Buehlmann (Switzerland)

Introduction

I work as a Solution Focused therapist, supervisor, coach, and trainer. I originally trained as a child and adolescent psychiatrist, but have also worked with adults in all areas for over 20 years. I am particularly fascinated by children and young people, as they always have such great ideas for solutions that we adults wouldn't even think of. The prerequisites for working in this context are listening well to children and young people and taking them seriously.

I would like to point out that the text can give the impression that there is a clear separation of the genders, as though only two genders exist (namely man and woman). I also work with people from the LBGTQ community, and I see there that the definition of gender is not so simple, and the transitions can also be fluid. For the sake of simplicity, however, I will limit myself to the female and male gender when answering the questions in the text.

Reflect on how your gender influences your work–life and being a Solution Focused practitioner

It is quite amazing that I have never asked myself this question before. There are several aspects to the question that run through my mind, one being how I see my gender directly influencing my working life and my work as a Solution Focused practitioner. Another is that women are generally said to have certain typical qualities of empathy (Christov-Moore et al., 2014), handle emotions well, show warmth in social interactions, have good listening skills, and are often self-critical. I am sceptical whether such generalisations can be made. Many men have these qualities too. To some extent, they can also be learned. I also recognise some of these qualities as part of my skills or personality. I think that I am a good listener and that I can put myself in other people's shoes well. I am also quite self-critical and try to question my actions again and again. These qualities may at some point have played a part in my decision to become a psychiatrist and psychotherapist.

Another aspect of this question is how my life as a woman, as a wife, and as a mother influences my work today. A joint agreement with my husband resulted in

DOI: 10.4324/9781003430254-10

me taking on a greater share of the housework and the care of our children in terms of time at the beginning of our family life. This resulted in me working part-time soon after entering the workforce, and thus influenced my career. Only when the children were older was I able to commit more time to my work and, as a result, international contacts and cooperation only came about later in my career. The search for a part-time job also brought me to Solution Focused work by chance in 1993, when I started working at an institution that was already using the Solution Focused approach. So, thank goodness for being a woman! Perhaps Solution Focusing also helped me, and still helps me, to better cope with the challenges of being a woman, a professional woman, a wife, and a mother of two grown-up children. The Solution Focused approach helps me to focus more on the positive, it enables me to ask questions professionally and in my private life instead of immediately having answers ready, to focus on resources even in difficult situations, and to appreciate what is already there.

In the everyday course of my practice, my gender certainly plays a role on another level. How do clients choose their therapist? Different factors such as availability and gender play a role, as do clients' cultural background, life history, and experience. When asked, one client said that she felt that a female therapist had similar experiences and thought patterns, and therefore she felt better understood. She felt safer with a woman. Therefore, only a female therapist would be an option for her. A young man said that he thought he could talk about feelings better with me as a woman than with a man.

Reflecting on gender and Solution Focused work, I noticed something else the other day: in our practice, where six women work, there are many pictures of flowers on the walls and there are always flowers on the tables. Are practice interiors different depending on whether men or women work in them? Do flowers belong more to female facilities? On the question of gender influence, I would like to conclude with a basic consideration, and that is that I believe gender differences are rather smaller than we assume. In psychotherapy, the relationship between client and therapist is very important, and that depends on many more factors than gender. Gender differences have more to do with education, socialisation, and social role attributions than with biology (Beck, 2014).

What is your good reason for staying a Solution Focused practitioner?

There are several reasons why I work as a Solution Focused therapist, supervisor, coach, and trainer. I like the approach, with its focus on what works, what succeeds, what resources there are, and the future that the client hopes for. Many of the basic assumptions are in line with my worldview; for example, that the client is knowledgeable and an expert on himself. Meeting clients at eye level and having mutual respect are very important to me. The Solution Focused approach frees me from the burden of having to be an expert or to create hypotheses. Instead, it allows me to be curious and ask questions with an interest in details about preferred futures and things already going well. Exploring resources with clients is also very satisfying for me. I have learned to trust the process of Solution Focused practice and have the experience to know that it works. Getting a lot of positive feedback from clients reinforces my belief that the Solution Focused approach is right for my work.

I like the different tools that the Solution Focused approach offers: best hopes and exception questions; scaling questions that can be used in so many ways; pre-assumptions that are made and are often so helpful when you're stuck, for example, "Let's say things got a little better tomorrow, what would be the first small sign you'd notice?" When working with children and young people, the Solution Focused approach fits well because children are curious by nature, they like to try out new things and are very creative in finding solutions. They learn through "trial and error" anyway. They don't want to analyse problems and, fortunately, they are not very surprised by miracles. Adolescents usually aim to get rid of the therapist as quickly as possible because they often do not come voluntarily but are sent by adults (Berg & Steiner, 2003). For them, the focus on a hoped-for future and resources usually fits very well and they are grateful that they don't have to focus on problems.

It is simply more fun to talk about solutions, best hopes, and preferred futures, about what has already succeeded and exceptions to problems, than to analyse problems. This is an important aspect of staying healthy as a counsellor (Medina & Beyebach, 2014), and in my private life. I also experience that working with a Solution Focused approach often brings about hoped-for changes quite quickly. And as a medical doctor, as a therapist, I feel obliged by the financial pressure and the pressure of demand in the healthcare system to try to work with people as briefly as possible.

What would others notice you doing that would tell them that you work from a Solution Focused approach?

My clients notice that, time and again, even when talking about problems and difficult, complex life situations, in addition to appreciating the burdens I also make the switch to questions about hoped-for changes, to what has already worked, and to resources. So, I always try to change the focus of clients with my questions, to expand the possibilities they can see. And, of course, to support them in bringing all the resources they have to the fore and making these available again. Perhaps it is also my way of listening, focusing on what clients offer in terms of solutions and resources – as Yvonne Dolan says, listening with a "third ear" (Dolan, 2013).

Even if I take the role of an expert for a moment during conversations, for example when clients want to talk about medication, there is always room for a Solution Focused question, such as, "Assuming the medication has exactly the effect you hope for, how would you know that it works well?" This is usually a surprising question for clients. Occasional expertise on the part of the therapist is thus embedded in the Solution Focused engagement, resulting in co-expertise between client and therapist.

My colleagues who work in a more problem-oriented way, and with whom I exchange ideas in team reflections, notice that I always ask questions that are rather unusual for them: for example, "How would your client notice that this case review was helpful? What exactly would you do differently?" And, not to forget, my husband at home notices that in the evening I usually talk about the sparkling moments of the day, even when the day has been very demanding.

Share an exercise that might be useful to other women practitioners

I learned the "Make the best of it" exercise from Terese Steiner (2016) at the Solution Focused World Conference in Amsterdam. You do the exercise in pairs.

- Each person makes a drawing of their choice on an A4 sheet of paper.
- Afterwards they exchange their drawings.
- Then the drawing of the other person has to be destroyed. Anything can be done with it, but the sheet has to remain whole.
- The drawings are swapped back.
- Each person is given the instruction, "And now make the best of it" (using their original drawing).

I use this exercise when one of the best hopes is formulated beforehand in conversation as, "I have to make the best of it". For example: I saw a young woman with inflammatory bowel disease. The disease caused her to question her whole life, she did not eat properly, and became very depressed. When asked about her best hopes for the conversation, one of the things she said was that she would succeed in making the best of the situation. In the conversation we worked out a lot of details about this. How exactly would she notice that she could make the best of it? What difference would it make to her, and who else would notice that she was succeeding? Then we did this exercise. The exercise is another way of experiencing what the client has previously articulated. Exercises are used differently by each therapist. How do you think you could use this exercise in your context?

Share how you adapt the approach and make it your own. Give us five characteristics that are a part of your Solution Focused DNA

I see the Solution Focused approach more as a meta-approach. I use helpful tools from different therapeutic or counselling directions in a Solution Focused way. These can be elements from Gestalt or hypnotherapy, or trauma therapy approaches such as resource and EMDR. The embedding of suggested exercises in Solution Focusing is done, for example, with the question, "Let's say this exercise we have done now is useful for you. How would you notice that?" (Buehlmann & Wheeler, 2018).

Since I work a lot with children and young people, I also adapt the approach to people who do not yet have fully developed language skills (Berg & Steiner, 2003). So, I offer more than talking, as solutions and resources can be experienced with all senses and the whole body during a conversation (Buehlmann & Wheeler, 2018). Besides co-constructing solutions through talking, there can also be the doing and experiencing of solutions and resources. For example, at the end of the first session, when we have talked about best hopes, miracles, or days "when things go a little better", I often let the clients choose a picture from a collection of images (Krause & Storch, 2018), asking them to choose one that fits their best hopes/miracles/ "things go a little better". They may also find a movement that goes with the picture, and a phrase or keyword. As Gunther Schmidt explained, experiences are big networks on different levels and in different brain regions, always connected with the body and in exchange with the environment (2016). This underpins the idea that solutions and resources can be experienced with all the senses and the whole body, in addition to talking. I offer this on the assumption that it creates new neuronal networks in the whole body that can trigger changes. This approach is not only appreciated by children and young people but has also proven its worth in work with adults.

I also see the Solution Focused approach in certain situations and contexts as a co-expertise of client and therapist/supervisor. Sometimes I share experiences and knowledge if the client asks for it, and I ask how it can be useful to him. As a medical doctor, occasionally I also take on an expert role when I discuss medication with clients. Here I can also remain Solution Focused as an expert, by informing them well and, of course, leaving the choice to the client, and by asking, for example, "Exactly how would you notice that the medicine works the way you hope?"

As a medical doctor, I often work also in a problem-oriented system. Reports to insurance companies, for example, are formulated in a completely different language to the language I use with clients. I have to explain this to clients and colleagues. I adapt my questions and my way of working to the context in which I am working. It makes a difference whether I am working with a young man who is completely withdrawn, who hears voices and feels persecuted, or whether I am coaching a woman who no longer feels comfortable in her professional environment and wants to realign herself. Despite such differences, something always stays the same no matter what the context – asking questions about a preferred future; asking about events from the past that have to do with the preferred future; talking about the next small steps; and focusing on the resources that will help the client to go his way into this future.

Which female practitioner inspires you and in which way?

Therese Steiner inspired me a lot and still does. She is a child and adolescent psychiatrist and comes from Zurich, Switzerland. She often worked with Insoo

Kim Berg and Steve de Shazer. Together with Insoo she wrote the book *Children's solution work* (Berg & Steiner, 2003). I have learned a lot from her, her books, and her videos. In my supervision with her it is helpful that she asks me questions that make me question my own constructions and ideas. Through her example I also find it easier to navigate tensions between the medical context with its rather problem-oriented approach and my Solution Focused work.

What soft small notion would you encourage other women practitioners to embrace?

I am convinced that every practitioner has exactly the right thoughts for herself. For myself, it has helped to work a lot with other colleagues, men and women, to learn from others, and thus to develop my own personal style.

My best hopes for other female Solution Focused voices

Ich hoffe und bin zuversichtlich, dass noch mehr Frauen als Dozentinnen, Hauptredner Innen, in Publikationen und Schlüsselstellen in Institutionen in Erscheinung treten Und so eine noch ausgeglichene Sichtweise in der Lösungsfokussierung Platz findet. Ich wünsche uns Frauen, dass wir voller Selbstvertrauen und mit grosser Offenheit auftreten. Die gegenseitige Unterstützung hilft dabei sehr.

I hope and am confident that even more women will appear as lecturers, keynote speakers, in publications, and in key positions in institutions. I also hope that an even more balanced view will find its way into the Solution Focused community. My wish is that all women show more self-confidence and more openness. Mutual support among one another is always helpful.

Author's reflection

Reflecting on how my gender influences my work has been very challenging. I know that my gender influences my work with clients, but how exactly? What would my clients say about it? Is there such a thing as gender bias? I have come to the conclusion that many other factors influence my work with clients as much as or more than gender. And I have reconsidered my own construction of differences between women and men. Are we really as different as we are often made out to be? I was also happy to notice how many female colleagues have accompanied me for years, how I could and still do learn a lot from them. I believe that female solidarity in the Solution Focused community is essential. I have become aware that with the Solution Focused approach I have found a way of working that fulfils me and that I still enjoy my work very much.

Co-constructive editors' reflection

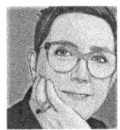

I was very grateful for Ursula challenging us in this chapter to think about our own assumptions about gender. Can we generalise and ascribe any qualities only to women? Maybe these qualities are not for women only? Maybe we should think more about the qualities of the profession rather than the qualities of gender. However, at the end of the chapter she does notice a soft touch of flowers on the table in her office, where only women work.

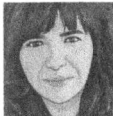

Yes, and this makes me think that even though she challenges the assumption that gender plays a specific role in how we work, she is also open to noticing the subtle differences it makes, nearly in an unconscious, underlying way. Yet, she does say that gender differences are less pronounced than we assume.

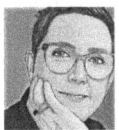

And I loved that she talked of gender being fluid and on a continuum, somewhere in between. In between male and female. I was also impressed that she asked her clients about how they felt gender influenced her practice and both her male and female clients said they preferred a female therapist because they thought women understood emotions better.

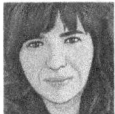

What really stood out for me about this chapter is how Ursula knows she works in a problem-saturated world and knows that as a medical doctor she sometimes has to be the "expert" prescribing a client medication; however, she is always mindful of taking a balanced view and shifting the conversation to possibility. I really liked that she constantly mentions how she is self-critical and aware of what she brings into the foreground.

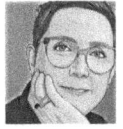

Yes, what's embedded in her practice is that you have to look at both sides. I also noticed her ability to be self-reflective and constantly aware of her actions and decisions. It is as though Ursula is reminding us to be on our toes all the time, that we always have to pay attention to the balance between problem talk and solution talk. We need to be mindful of creating an interference, find the cracks that make a small disturbance, and allow hope and possibility in.

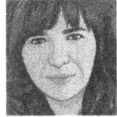

Yes, exactly. We need to constantly be aware of creating pattern interruptions in the problem narrative. She says it is our job to switch the focus and this requires concentration and focus on the part of the practitioner. She also mentions that constantly shifting focus is good and healthy for both client and practitioner. This reminds me of the idea of vicarious resilience, which helps us see ourselves and our clients in a more hopeful and positive light (Froerer & von Cziffra-Bergs, 2018).

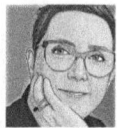

Yes, there is so much evidence of this, for example, the work by Mark Beyenbach et al. (2018), which shows that when you work in a Solution Focused way you are less burnt out, less overwhelmed and stressed, and have more energy because you give back ownership to the client. I also loved what Ursula said about adolescents and mandated clients and how she focuses on a hopeful future. She calls all her clients co-experts in the process, which I loved because it already makes the client competent.

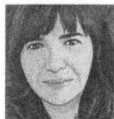

Yes, and if you want to co-construct a solution you use a co-expert to help you. I always think of the client's strengths as my co-therapist; however, Ursula sees the client as a co-expert in the whole process.

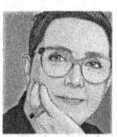

What really stood out for me is that Ursula mentions that the Solution Focused approach is a meta-approach for her and that she will adapt any other idea or technique to suit her meta-approach, all in the best interest of her client. Ursula uses the Solution Focused approach as her umbrella, and she integrates other elements creatively and makes it her own.

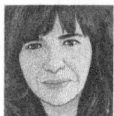

Yes, it is like rainwater that seeps into everything she does and becomes a personal philosophy, stance, and way of being present in life, which reminds me of the *being* Solution Focused and how it influences not only her professional life but also her personal life. I find it so inspirational to talk about it as a meta-approach because it allows us all to have our own Solution Focused style, our own *being, doing and experiencing* that influence our actions, feelings, and behaviours. The elements of other approaches that Ursula integrates into her work are still grounded in the Solution Focused assumptions.

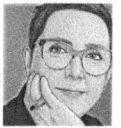

I also loved that she mentioned that children are not surprised by miracles. This made me think that if we do not play with miracles and imagine, then we miss a huge opportunity to create change with a child because they already live in imagine-land. And that she ends her chapter inviting other practitioners to use this approach with more confidence and openness, almost as though she is giving us all permission to use it in our own unique ways. She challenges us in a gentle and subtle way to look at our own assumptions and beliefs and gently highlights that there is already a lot going right in our field and that we need to pay attention to that.

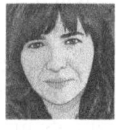

Her chapter is like a boomerang bringing us right back to ourselves, reminding us to be mindful of our assumptions and pay attention to what is already working and going well.

Author references

Beck, H. (2014). *Hirnrissig*. Hanser.

Berg, I., & Steiner, T. (2003). *Children's solution work*. Norton.

Beyebach, M., Neipp, M.C., García, M., & González, I. (2018). Impact of nurses' Solution-Focused communication on the fluid adherence of adult patients on haemodialysis. *Journal of Advanced Nursing, 74*, 2654–2657. https://doi.org/10.1111/jan.13792

Buehlmann, U., & Wheeler, J. (2018). Going beyond words. In T. Switek, B. Strahilov & P. Panayotov (Eds.), *Making waves: Solution Focused practice in Europe* (pp. 171–191). PIK-BS.

Christov-Moore, L., Simpson, E., Coudéb, G., Grigaitytea, K., Iacobonia, M., & Ferrari, P. (2014). Empathy: Gender effects in brain and behavior. *Neurosci Biobehav Rev., 46*(4), 604–627.

Dolan, Y. (2013, September 30). *"It seemed so simple in the beginning"* [Paper presentation]. EBTA One Day Post Conference Workshop, Bern, Switzerland.

Krause, F., & Storch, M. (2018). *Ressourcen aktivieren mit dem Unbewussten*. ZRM Bildkartei. Hogrefe.

Medina, A., & Beyebach, M. (2014). The impact of Solution-Focused training on professionals' beliefs, practices and burnout of child protection workers in Tenerife Island. *Child Care in Practice, 20*(1), 7–36.

Schmidt, G. (2016, 28 May). "Reden reicht nicht" [Conference]. Heidelberg, Germany.

Steiner, T. (2016, 11 June). *Skills and solution* [Conference session]. SF World Conference, Amsterdam, Netherlands.

Editor references

Antonio, M., Beyebach, M., & García, F.E. (2022). Effectiveness and cost-effectiveness of a solution-focused intervention in child protection services. *Journal of Children and Youth Services Review 143*(4). https://www.sciencedirect.com/science/article/pii/S01907 40922003395

Froerer, A., & von Cziffra-Bergs, J. (2018). Vicarious resilience. In A. Froerer, J. von Cziffra-Bergs, J. Kim & E. Connie (Eds.), *Solution Focused Brief Therapy and clients managing trauma* (pp. 226–235). Oxford University Press.

Chapter 10

Finding hope
Solution Focused work with traumatised and underprivileged clients

Dragana Knezić (Croatia)

Introduction

I work with refugees, torture and trauma survivors, and other people struggling to achieve their basic rights and live a dignified life. I work with the forgotten. The Solution Focused approach has transformed my practice with clients who have difficult lives and survived the most traumatic life events. The Solution Focused approach has equipped me with the stance and skills to be a more hopeful and optimistic helper.

Reflect on how your gender influences your work–life and being a Solution Focused practitioner

For most of my career I have been working in non-governmental organisations (NGOs) as a psychologist, counsellor, and human rights advocate. These roles are intertwined and inseparable to me, in the context of my professional and personal development in the post-conflict, transitional countries that emerged after the dissolution of the former Yugoslavia.

I am privileged that many remarkable, independent women have influenced me. My mother was the first woman in her family to work outside the household and earn a salary. She brought up two daughters and did almost all the household work in our family. She did not impose expectations on me and my sister to fulfil traditional female roles such as getting married (while still young), having children, raising them, and caring for elderly parents. In fact, she guarded us against such expectations from others in our community. In that sense, she was quite successful and both of us followed less traditional paths. The only thing we could expect her to be disappointed about would be if we weren't better educated than she was or were financially dependent on the men in our lives.

The women who inspired me while I was a psychology student and early on in my career were on the forefront of the anti-war movement and founded NGOs that still promote and protect human rights and support disadvantaged individuals and groups. My career followed a similar path and I started working with refugee children and youth during and in the aftermath of the Yugoslavian war.

DOI: 10.4324/9781003430254-11

Later I continued to work with other vulnerable beneficiaries, mostly those affected by societal and economic transformations.

I have witnessed how women like my mother were the first to lose their jobs in an economic transition, as a rule without fair compensation or opportunities to find new employment; how they had to find a way to provide for their family when their husbands became redundant; how it is so much harder for women who are victims of a war crime to get justice, reparation, and public sympathy without judgement. As I was brought up to feel equal to anyone, to know that I can match anyone in terms of competence and effort, and not to be bound to any role I do not choose, I became increasingly sensitive to the inequalities and injustices faced by women and others deprived of equal opportunities. A sense of solidarity and drive to act in accordance with my beliefs led me to a career in public service and at NGOs, where I feel I can help to reduce inequalities and empower the underprivileged.

During my career I have almost always been surrounded, supported, and inspired by women helpers, activists, and volunteers. Many of them stand up for their beliefs, defending principles and advocating for the oppressed at the cost of being undermined, disparaged, ridiculed, or even threatened, usually based on their gender. In a society that is re-examining its fundamental values in the aftermath of a war and socio-economic transition, active non-compliance with the traditional perspective on gender and the role of women in public life has become part of my professional and personal identity, as it did for my role models.

As a female Solution Focused practitioner, I am constantly aware of systemic disadvantages standing in the way of my beneficiaries living the best lives they can. So, I have one foot in Solution Focused practice, employing a "not-knowing stance" (de Jong & Berg, 2013) while working with beneficiaries, and one foot in envisaging and co-constructing solutions, "having an agenda" for the community and society in which I work and live.

What is your good reason for staying a Solution Focused practitioner?

Working in the field of rehabilitation of torture and trauma survivors I have come to know the devastating, long-term and pervasive effects such experiences have on survivors, their families, and communities; the transgenerational transfer of trauma and how it contributes to the vicious cycle of violence in societies torn apart by ethnic, religious. or racial conflicts. The recent history of my country(ies) provides sufficient evidence and examples. As problem-oriented approaches still dominate in this field, I was taught that the path to recovery leads through a detailed and in-depth account of the traumatic event and re-experiencing related emotions in the safety of the psychotherapeutic process (Basoglu, 1992; Herman, 2015). Inevitably, this is, in my experience, painful for the survivor, disheartening for the therapist, and requires time – that irreplaceable resource. I often felt ineffective and discouraged as a helper. Yet I learned about and met people who seemed to live productive, fulfilling lives regardless of their lived traumatic experiences; individuals who managed to transform the painful historical trauma of their ancestors through their own peace activism. Problem-oriented approaches did not satisfyingly account for these exceptions that seemed so important to me.

It was a lucky coincidence that I discovered the Solution Focused approach while looking for something different that could help our small team at the Rehabilitation Centre for Stress and Trauma to effectively and efficiently face the challenge of a growing number of refugees coming to Europe from war-torn countries in the Middle East who need support to recover from traumatic experiences and move on with their lives in a new environment. The Solution Focused approach equipped me with a stance, attitudes, and skills consistent with my hopes for the role of helper. I learned how to carefully and attentively listen for and reflect back to survivors their strengths, abilities, skills, and "small acts of resistance" (Wade, 1997), while empathetically and patiently acknowledging their suffering and pain, if they chose to share that story with me. This has made me a more trustful, hopeful, and optimistic helper. It deeply moves me each time I notice when a client who has suffered and survived horrific experiences starts to hope and shows confidence in her capacity to achieve what she hopes for, when gently asked about it. Working with clients towards what they want to be different in their lives, and only that, is both respectful to the client and heartening for the helper. This effortlessly and naturally gives back control and autonomy to the survivor, which is a universal postulate of trauma recovery.

Not holding on to assumptions and hypotheses about clients' problems or the criteria that constitutes their recovery is very liberating. The old programme that was running in the background of my conversations with the client has been uninstalled, leaving me with free processing capacities to engage profoundly in listening and connecting with the client and her story, discovering remarkable exceptions that are useful.

What would others notice you doing that would tell them that you work from a Solution Focused approach?

The clients I work with already notice the difference in my curiosity about what they want and my acceptance that this is what they need in the way I acknowledge without questioning their account of the difficulties they are dealing with or their experience of the institutional setting they have encountered (de Jong & Berg, 2013). They might notice I am both listening attentively and empathetically to their account of their suffering and struggles and hearing and reflecting on every notion of success or coping. I hope that gives them the sense they are heard and respected, and at the same time encouraged.

Other helpers I work with notice that I approach clients who have had harsh life experiences with hope and optimism, trust, and amazement about their ability to cope, survive, and, at the very least, have hopes for the future.

My fellow activists notice that I am more interested in finding out how we want things to be different than in all that is wrong in our society and who is to blame. They might notice that I notice and encourage others to notice and celebrate our successes, however small; even the slightest changes leading to the equality and justice we are envisioning; that I am taking every opportunity to highlight our contribution to progressive social change.

Share an exercise that might be useful to other practitioners

This is an exercise I learned from Dr Stephen Langer (during the workshop "Application of Solution Focused Brief Approach in Mentoring", held in Croatia in 2018). I often use it in different variations in group work. It is particularly useful for groups that work together or know each other well, such as the groups of volunteers helping refugees and undocumented migrants that I occasionally support. I ask a group member to name one of her superpowers and how she notices she is using that superpower in her work or everyday life. Then I ask the other participants to give an account of when they noticed that superpower in action, what the person did exactly, and what the outcome was. The exercise proceeds with each member of the group discussing their superpower. It is a powerful way to build team cohesion, trust, and mutual support. Teams often report back that they continue to notice and give each other feedback on the plentiful evidence of competence, ability, resourcefulness, and strength that each member brings to the team. It is very useful in teams that set high standards for themselves and work in demanding settings on intensive tasks, as volunteers and activists usually do. When outside or professional support is lacking, this facilitates support and care from within the person and the team.

Share how you adapt the approach and make it your own. Give us five characteristics that are a part of your Solution Focused DNA

As I am relatively new to the approach, I find confidence in being a Solution Focused purist (Durrant, 2016) and strive to stick to the fundamental assumptions and strategies of the approach, as I learned it and as described in the seminal literature (De Shazer & Dolan, 2017; Pichot & Dolan, 2003; de Jong & Berg, 2013).

In 2016, when I started learning and practising the Solution Focused approach, Dr Stephen Langer and I developed *Short-term Solution Focused group intervention for refugee torture survivors* (Langer & Knezić, 2020) which was piloted as a part of an EU-funded project in three European countries. Jumping into the deep end of the pool and practising the consistent application of Solution Focused principles in challenging environments has empowered me. I now regularly apply the Solution Focused approach in different groups – counselling groups and support groups for foster parents, single-parent families, volunteers, and activists. I apply the Solution Focused principles and strategies in educational workshops on different topics, combining it with interactive exercises from an experiential learning toolkit.

Traumatised clients and those experiencing oppression, poverty, and marginalisation have taught me to exercise patience and deep empathy with their problem-saturated description, sometimes at the expense of brevity. I trust their good reasons for wanting to share detailed accounts of suffering and pain. The more such clients are convinced of my compassion and sense that they have been heard, the more genuinely they will accept and co-construct with the questions about exceptions I notice and reflect back to them.

I find that paying close attention and immediately co-constructing around exceptions fit my personal style and keep the Solution Focused conversation unfolding naturally with clients who are overwhelmed with the intensity and persistence of their problems. Noticing and focusing the conversation on exceptions, I believe, helps to cast light on their own agency and what's realistic in the circumstances of their life and our work.

Giving authentic and heartfelt compliments is something I particularly enjoy and do not spare throughout a Solution Focused conversation. When they are genuine and evidence-based, clients report that compliments stay with them and boost their confidence in their ability to achieve their hopes. In groups I use different exercises and tasks encouraging participants to notice each other's successes and give evidence-based compliments.

The Solution Focused approach has transformed both my work as helper and activist and how I approach my own life difficulties and important relationships. It helps me keep in focus what I want to be different and the small steps that are getting me there, instead of dwelling on problems. More importantly, I am more aware of how my actions invite interactions with persons I care about or respect, and lead to constructive, respectful relationships. I can see how anger, pride, hurt, blame, or self-pity, although still there occasionally, take a back seat to the sincere effort for life to be better.

Which female practitioner inspires you and in which way?

Living and working in a Solution Focused blind spot, in the Balkans, I have had to resort to training opportunities abroad and to books. The first book I read, after the introductory Solution Focused workshop, was Yvonne Dolan and Teri Pichot's *Solution-Focused Brief Therapy: Its effective use in agency settings*. It gave me a master recipe, just as Yvonne suggested in the first chapter of the book. Reading the book, I felt that I got it and I could do it! I found later that "getting it" is easy and that doing it consistently and effortlessly requires a lot of discipline and practice. But the way the approach is described and demonstrated in this book, the simplicity, straightforwardness, and practicality it suggested, possibly played a critical role in me getting hooked on and sticking with learning the Solution Focused practice. What inspired me as well was the warmth, compassion, and respectful acknowledgment of the difficulties the mandated clients experience in their encounters with agencies and of the good reasons they have for their behaviours and choices in the harsh circumstances of their lives. This tapped into my basic assumptions about disadvantaged people and was different from what I had been taught previously.

Insoo Kim Berg continues to inspire through her legacy. Reading the transcripts or listening to the recordings of her sessions, I was amazed at her compassion and kindness, which I am doing my best to emulate with my clients as well. And what inspires me the most is the effortlessness and flexibility with which she navigates the conversation. It seems to me she trusted her good Solution Focused judgement and the client: she was not bound by the linear progression through the stages of the work but rather "leading from one step behind" (de Jong & Berg, 2013) with flexibility and firm meandering.

Finally, my friend, colleague, and the only other Solution Focused practitioner in Croatia, Sandra Šipka, inspires me on many levels. She often challenges me with her divergent thinking, creativity, and intuitiveness. Working with her, I have learned there are many creative ways of expression to substitute or complement verbal communication; that not only are there different paths to an outcome but it is also possible to be happy with and enjoy diverse outcomes; and that making the journey can be as important and joyful as reaching the destination.

What soft small notion would you encourage other women practitioners to embrace?

After a workshop on the application of the Solution Focused approach in crisis intervention, one of the participants in her feedback stated that she valued my authenticity in presenting and facilitating. This compliment sticks with me, although it is not directly related to the usefulness of the content, exercises, process, or any other "material" component of the workshop, but rather to my characteristics, the presenter. I inferred that this compliment implied that the ideas I was presenting and the way I presented were an expression of my true self (Varga & Guignon, 2020). We are influenced by all our life experiences, direct and mediated encounters, what we have learned, including the Solution Focused approach, and what we need to unlearn. All those experiences and elements are blended in a unique way. I would like to encourage women practitioners to stay true to their own personality, spirit, and character, as the word authentic implies, while remaining firmly rooted in the fundamental Solution Focused assumptions and values; to behave and interact naturally in a Solution Focused conversation, as it feels comfortable and consistent with personal style. I would encourage women practitioners to trust and use their good sense. Finally, I would like to see women practitioners, particularly at the beginning of their careers, being kinder and more generous to themselves, their decisions and their mistakes.

My best hopes for other female Solution Focused voices

Nadam se da će nas, koje primjenjujemo Rješenjem Usmjereni pristup i koristimo se zajedničkim jezikom, biti puno više. Da ćemo brojnošću, organiziranošću, dosljednošću u primjeni Rješenjem Usmjerenog pristupa, kvalitetom i rezultatima ostaviti trag i postaviti nove standarde u pomagačkim profesijama. Nadam se da ćemo se međusobno podržavati, ohrabrivati i osnaživati, po tome biti prepoznatljive i time privlačiti nove generacije stručnjakinja.

I hope there will be many of us, speaking our common language, who are trained and who use the Solution Focused approach in different areas. That we will, in numbers, make a mark and set new standards in helping professions showing how well we are organised and how consistent we are in applying the Solution Focused approach. I hope we will support, encourage, and empower each other and that we will be known by these attributes and actions to the next generations of female practitioners.

Co-constructive editors' reflections

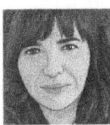

I loved how she answered the first question with such a strong voice for vulnerable and sensitive women. Dragana tells us that she does not only stand up for women and fight for women, but that she is also inspired by women.

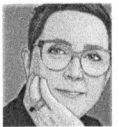

And, you know, telling the story about her mother, she was taking us back, which was wonderful. And I got the feeling that her mother was like, you know, the first feminist ever. A really strong woman. And that was fascinating to read about. In answering the first question, she shares how women who have been affected by war inspire her. She shares their hardship, how women lose their jobs during wartime, how they find themselves in bad situations, how a war context can affect a woman's life economically, culturally, and socially. I think that, both through her history and in her work life, Dragana has experienced these effects in so many contexts.

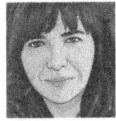

And Anne-Marie, she has seen that injustice. She has seen the hardship and the deep, terrible, harsh situations. I love it when she says that she has a building agenda when it comes to women. It's not only an empathic co-construction – she wants to build women up!

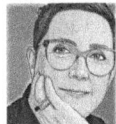

Yeah. She's on a mission. That is so clear. And I've been with Dragana a couple of times, and that is what I experienced too. This is so strong within her. The injustices that not only women but a lot of other people too have experienced. I was smiling when I read how individuals manage to transform painful trauma – that was what you and I talked about just the other day, this shift in language, and from now on and forever I will hold onto this when I work with traumatised people. They are people who have managed trauma!

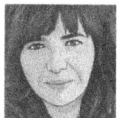

People who have managed trauma, yes, because the word presupposes coping and managing. And what I loved here, and she says it so beautifully, is that she is not going to get hooked on trauma experiences. And I know for me, in the book with Adam, Johnny, and Elliot, I wrote that I don't debrief trauma, I rebrief resilience. And this is the first woman, the first time anywhere I've read of somebody who gets it. Who's saying the very same thing, you know! Of course, we need to acknowledge, validate, and listen to the trauma experience, but it's very important to debrief that resilience, those coping skills, those competencies. And what Dragana does she does gently, which I love, she is not in a rush, she is patient and listens with gentle care, but she is always going to rebrief resilience.

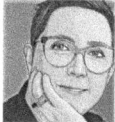

And I'm impressed by how far Dragana has come in a short period of time. She's saying, "I'm pretty new to Solution Focused thinking", yet she has already embedded the approach and taken so many different aspects of it into her practice, into her life, into her being. I rarely read about practitioners who are familiar with Dr Allan Wade, but I just did. Small acts of resistance, that is what it's all about.

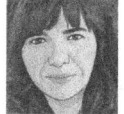

Agreed. She's like a sponge that just takes the Solution Focused words and ideas and soaks it all up, and then builds with it.

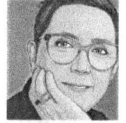

Yeah, that's right. And she writes about how others would notice that she is curious. I get the idea that she is curious not only about the Solution Focused approach but also about people in general. She has this curiosity that runs like a golden thread through this chapter.

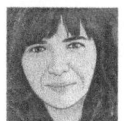

Anne-Marie, she doesn't question their difficulties, she is just curious about how they survived. And then, what I found brilliant is that she also doesn't question their best hopes. She's completely accepting of what the client thinks is best for them and not what her best hopes are for them.

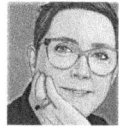

And that is really difficult sometimes. Easy to understand, but maybe not easy to do. What makes it quite difficult is to put yourself aside and really take a not-knowing position, which includes not having ideas about what is best for people, what their best hope should be.

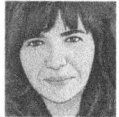

If you're on this mission to help people, and especially if you are working with people who are in really hard, difficult circumstances, to be able to put yourself totally aside and trust that they know what they want and that what they say they need is best for them is incredibly inspirational because that is not easy.

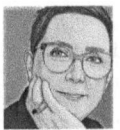

I was also inspired by the part where Dragana talks about approaching clients with hope and optimism. That is just beautiful, you know. Everybody, with or without a harsh life experience, is met with hope and optimism and that is beautiful. Also when she writes about her fellow activists, who might notice that she encourages others to notice and celebrate their successes. This is interweaving and interactional flow, and using what is between the noses is just beautiful.

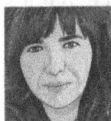

Dragan is so good at grounding everybody's experience; she validates and acknowledges and then she is very aware of exceptions and looks for tiny exceptions. It makes me think of Linda Metcalf, who wrote that exceptions are the bread and butter of the Solution Focused approach. And Dragana knows that, right, she really searches for those tiny exceptions in all the conversations. And she says when you keep looking for it, the conversation will unfold naturally.

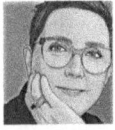

That is right. And she's sharing this exercise on superpowers. It's very inspiring, as I've realised there are so many ways of supporting or doing an exercise like this, you know? To visualise the superpower or to have a picture of the superpower or to draw the superpower. So, it's a very inspiring exercise for me.

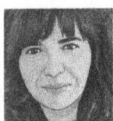

Yes, especially if you think about the context in which she works, where people feel they have no power, and then to notice their own superpower. She also tells people to watch the superpowers emerge. This is also a presupposition because she is saying superpowers are there, just search for them and they will be there, you have a superpower no matter what has happened to you.

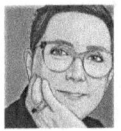

I was fascinated when Dragana said that, as a relatively new practitioner, she found confidence in being a Solution Focused purist. And I realised that I need to read Durrant's article. And that is what this project also brings to me, you know, so much inspiration about references and literature I still haven't read. For that I'm deeply grateful.

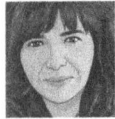

So brave, so courageous. It is as though she is pushing up her sleeves and saying, "Come, let's get going. Let's use this and help people." And there were some things Dragana said that I really could relate to. Like, the Balkans is a Solution Focused blind spot. Same with me here at the bottom of Africa. I also just had to use it, make it up and jump in and go for it, because you're actually doing it on your own. I was so impressed by her courage. Yes, just going for it.

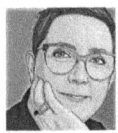

Yeah. That is a mission again. And then she is still a Solution Focused purist. She is developing her personal style and exceptions, finding her own personal style. It's not like she's just copy– pasting. No, no.

She has her personal style based on her lifelong experience in this field of working with refugees and traumatised or tortured people.

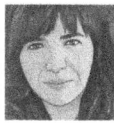

And with a strong focus on, "I'm doing it for a good reason". Something that she said a little bit later that really struck me was that she related to compassion and kindness as things that meander. And I love that word meandering, because again, it's that flexible flow of leading from behind. And it reminds me that she is so aware that conversations are a weaving process, a meandering process, not a linear process. I loved that.

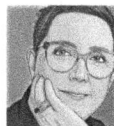

Yeah. Flexibly and firmly meandering. That is really nice.

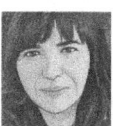

And again, that is a beautiful metaphor. It's a meander, you know, it's like a little stream that meanders through the forest. You know, it isn't a linear conversation full of techniques.

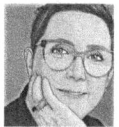

She has been pretty much on her own in a country where there are not many practitioners, if any. What impresses me is that it is a little bit harder to learn when you're on your own and don't have anybody to practise with. You only have books and tapes to rely on. And the impact that Yvonne Dolan and Terri Pichot's book had on her is so inspiring, and that she felt, "I get this and I can do this".

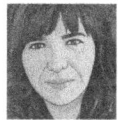

And then later on, she said that she learned that she also had to unlearn things. In order to be true to herself, in order to get it and do it, to use it in her own style with her own spirit and character, she needed to unlearn certain things.

And then there is the DNA, you know, I thought that was really beautiful. With that compliment about her presenting style she experienced that she was her true self. And isn't that what we all are aiming to be.

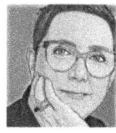

And again, she's not only encouraging us all to bring that out and make it our own style where we feel comfortable and consistent. Dragana is so adamant about being authentic and our true self that she even gives us what it means in the dictionary. This is such a beautiful hope for women, and it reminded me of what she wrote in the beginning on how women have to work that much harder because of the injustices and the difficulties of their struggle. We just have to be kinder and more generous to ourselves.

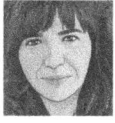

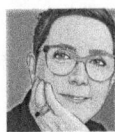

And we don't have to hit ourselves on the head each time we make a mistake, because we all make mistakes, a lot of mistakes, and it's okay, we do not need to have a bad conscience about it. We have to be gentle and embrace ourselves – our mistakes and our decisions. Some of them are good, some of them are not, but we don't have to blame ourselves all the time. And I thought, if I have to pick some sentences for the book's back cover this would be one of them: "I would like to see women being kinder and more generous to themselves, their decisions and their mistakes".

Author references

Basoglu, M. (Ed.). (1992). *Torture and its consequences: Current treatment approaches.* Cambridge University Press.

De Jong P., & Berg I.K. (2013). *Interviewing for solutions* (4th ed., instructor's). Brooks/Cole Cengage Learning.

De Shazer, S., & Dolan, Y. (2017). *More than miracles. The state of the art of Solution Focused Brief Therapy.* Routledge.

Durrant, M. (2016). Confessions of an unashamed Solution-Focused purist: What is (and isn't) Solution-Focused? *Journal of Solution Focused Practices, 2*(1).

Herman, J. (2015). *Trauma and recovery: The aftermath of violence – from domestic abuse to political terror.* Basic Books.

Langer, S.M., & Knezić, D. (2020). Short-term Solution Focused group intervention for refugee torture survivors. In K. Dierolf, D. Hogan, S. Hoorn & S. Wignaraja (Eds.), *Solution Focused practice around the world* (pp. 171–178). Routledge.

Merriam-Webster. (n.d.). *Authentic.* Merriam-Webster.com. https://www.merriam-webster.com/dictionary/authentic

Pichot, T., & Dolan, Y.M. (2003). *Solution-Focused Brief Therapy: Its effective use in agency settings.* Routledge.

Varga, S., & Guignon, C. (2020). *Authenticity.* Stanford Encyclopaedia of Philosophy. https://plato.stanford.edu/entries/authenticity/#RecAccAut

Wade, A. (1997). Small acts of living: Everyday resistance to violence and other forms of oppression. *Contemporary Family Therapy, 19*, 23–39.

Editor reference

Metcalf, L. (2009). Solution Focused therapy: Its applications and opportunities. In E. Connie & L. Metcalf (Eds.), *The art of Solution Focused therapy.* Springer Publishing.

Chapter 11

Solution Focused embodiment practice for empowerment

Olga Zotova (Russia)

Introduction

I am a coach, psychotherapist, embodiment facilitator, and trainer from Moscow, Russia. In 2022 I moved to Tel Aviv, Israel, but I continue working online with Russian and international clients. I view life as a process where body, mind, and culture are interconnected and I believe that understanding what is happening on a non-verbal and intersubjective level can be a valuable source of insight. This integrative perspective allows me to be creative and find diverse ways for "doing more of what works". What helps me to stay hopeful in this work, despite the current political situation in my home country, is my unwavering belief in people's resilience. It is rewarding to witness clients, who initially felt stuck, tap into their strengths and community support, and to see their sense of agency grow.

Reflect on how your gender influences your work–life and being a Solution Focused practitioner

My journey into the field of psychotherapy began together with my motherhood. Before that I worked in advertising and HR, in a business culture that didn't emphasise the significance of female experience. My motherhood allowed me to see the self-evident aspects of women's lives that were once invisible to me. For several years, together with my friend Alfiya Rakhmanova, I led dance movement groups called BabyContact (Rakhmanova, 2010) for mothers with infants and toddlers, focusing on the mother–baby relationship and co-presence. Reflecting on this work, I realised how important it was to create a space of friendly acceptance, a place where women could overcome social isolation, get away from daily chores, experience their time with the baby as precious, and share their difficulties with others in similar situations.

Later on, while working with women as a therapist, I noticed that qualities and activities that are traditionally considered "female" tend to be neglected or even marginalised.

This process occurs on multiple levels:

DOI: 10.4324/9781003430254-12

- In society, women often face such obstacles as discrimination, gender stereo-types, sexual harassment, gender pay gap, and a lack of representation in decision-making positions. In their families, they often experience silencing and the invisibility of "labour of care". Such attitudes can then be internal-ised by women themselves, causing them to undervalue their qualities and the efforts they make.
- On a psychological level, modalities such as emotions, feelings, and sensations, or qualities such as care and intuition, are frequently overlooked in favour of rational thinking and actions.
- Even in therapy training we can see an excessive focus on techniques at the expense of more foundational factors such as empathy, presence, and thera-peutic alliance. This is despite decades of research and meta-analysis confirm-ing the critical role these factors play in successful therapy outcomes (Duncan et al., 2010).

While overcoming these obstacles, women develop unique skills in coping and self-organisation, but these skills often remain unnoticed. Aided critical reflection and formulation of personal values can lead to women's empowerment.

I believe women themselves should take the lead in making the world a more sup-portive place, consciously using their unique knowledge and perspectives such as cooperation, acceptance, and care. Helping professionals could enhance this by creating accessible formats that promote social support and exchange of implicit knowledge.

What is your good reason for staying a Solution Focused practitioner?

When I began to work as a corporate coach, I was immediately inspired by the ideas and tools of Solution Focused coaching. It felt very suitable and resonated with my own values. Sticking to the ideas of Solution Focused therapy is my way to maintain hope, even in the most dire situations. It has taught me where to look for people's strengths and exclusions from their problem story. It also fosters cre-ativity: "If something doesn't work, try something different" is not just a slogan for me – it is the guiding principle that I put into practice.

I like the practicality of the approach. The idea of moving in small steps and noticing small signs of what is already present now (I call it "preferred future-in-the-present") facilitates connections between "landscape of identity" and "land-scape of action", between a new perception and a person's day-to-day reality.

This perspective helps me to see the person as someone possessing resources, strengths, and values, even if it is not (yet!) visible to the person themselves.

What would others notice you doing that would tell them that you work from a Solution Focused approach?

First of all, they would notice that I attune and listen. Then they would notice that I can be different with different clients, flexibly matching techniques to the person.

They would notice me doing the scaling frequently, sometimes in very creative ways. For me it is not just a technique; it is the way to transform yes/no, black-and-white thinking into a process of becoming. Scaling is my way to practise acceptance of the person the way they are. As Carl Rogers said, "The curious paradox is that when I accept myself just as I am, then I can change" (Rogers, 1995).

Once we agree on the spectrum of the scale, it feels easier to explore what the person has already accomplished to land at the current point on the scale. Thus, in a simple way, it conveys my attitude: that I am okay with whatever "number" they are at the moment.

Seen from the outside, the Solution Focused approach can seem very goal-oriented. While it is indeed a great coaching tool, it doesn't have to be pushy. As John Henden, a British Solution Focused therapist, so often points out, we are Solution Focused, not solution forced (Henden, 2014).

The lack of an extensive theoretical vocabulary eliminates the need to pigeon-hole the client inside the model and allows me to remain closer to the phenomeno-logical reality of my clients – and to speak their language. The idea of a preferred future is not an easy concept to handle. For ages the unknown has been perceived by humans as threatening, triggering our stress response and leading to feelings of anxiety or fear. The Solution Focused toolkit enables both therapists and clients to look into the unknown without a sense of threat but rather with curiosity and anticipation.

Share an exercise that might be useful to other women practitioners

Embodying "my support community"

Nobody travels through their life journey alone; fellow beings accompany us and make a contribution to our preferred set of values. By recognising their contribu-tion we can enhance our connection to these values, thus becoming more resilient to stress and hardships.

This exercise complements this idea with embodiment practice (Palmer & Crawford, 2013).

Step 1 – imagining your challenge in front of you: this could be a challenging or stress-ful situation at work, or a difficult conversation ahead. Now, notice: how does that impact your body? Just observe any sensations, feelings, and thoughts that arise. If there is any tension, try to determine where exactly and how you sense it.

Step 2 – putting together your "support community": take a sheet of paper and write down the names of potential members of your "support community". Who could be part of your support team in this situation (real people, imaginary fig-ures, fictional characters, pets, etc.)? The list doesn't have to be long; just make sure there are at least some figures on it.

Step 3 – embodying your "support community": now, imagine this team standing by your side in the challenging situation. Where exactly would you like to place

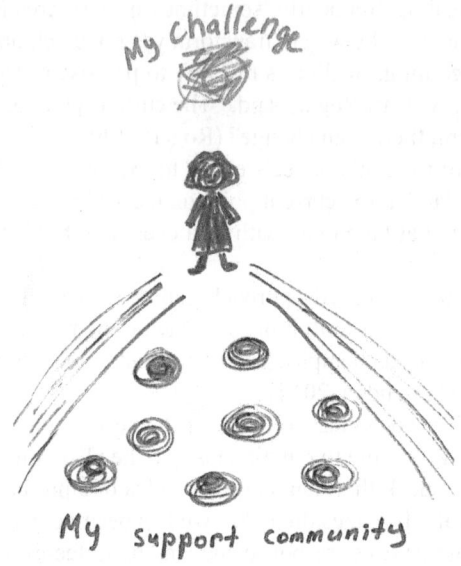

Figure 11.1 My support community

your team (behind you, "covering your back", or on the side)? Immerse yourself for a while in the experience that there are characters, real and imaginary, who share your values and aspirations and support you.

Now notice: how is your initial situation perceived from this state of bodymind (any difference in sensations, feelings, thoughts, the way you perceive yourself and the world)?

Step 4 – holding on to the sense of the "support community": if you find this state valuable, take some time to think about what could help you to maintain it and/ or connect with it when needed (it could be an image of the people on your "team", or a keyword, a movement, or a body posture).

It may be helpful to develop a micro-practice out of this, for example, taking a few deep breaths and imagining your "support team" standing by your side, or saying keywords to remind yourself of their support. Find what works best for you and use it when you need it.

Share how you adapt the approach and make it your own. Give us five characteristics that are a part of your Solution Focused DNA

Collaboration: my work is based on the principle of cooperation, so we decide together where to go, what topic to work on, and in what way. The more complicated the situation is, the more temptation there is to put on an "expert" hat and start telling people how to live their lives. But the hardship has already made people lose their agency and feel like the victims of their problems, so if we echo that, we will just be doing more of what doesn't work. These fundamental values of the Solution Focused approach as a non-expert position and the ethics of collaboration can function as an inoculation against what I call "method-centred therapy" and help us to step aside and listen.

Integration: my approach has been integrative from the beginning. My starting point on the journey to psychotherapy was dance movement therapy, which focuses on the integrity of body and mind as an inseparable part of who we are. I was strongly influenced by the liberating concepts of narrative practice, which directs our attention to the social context and the discourses that influence us, while providing a variety of tools for community work. I also learnt to work with trauma using Eye Movement Desensitisation and Reprocessing (EMDR), which focuses on the integration of traumatic memories held in the bodymind. Thus, I was bound to develop my own way of integrating different methods. The principles of Solution Focused therapy provide a perfect theoretical and methodological framework for this.

Embodiment (attention to the non-verbal, implicit level): I believe that we are grounded in the wholeness of the body–mind–culture–nature, so different layers of being continuously influence each other. Even without applying bodymind techniques directly, when listening to the client, I try to stay attentive to non-verbal language and embodied states. This can help me to better attune and notice subtle changes in breathing, body posture, or facial expression that could mark the transition from "problem land" to "solution land". Having noticed a subtle change, I can then ask a question about it. Our embodiment is the quickest way to travel to a preferred future because we can get there immediately. When we work with the body, "miracle" is always within reach: it is the miracle of the change of state.

Awareness of social context: I find it essential to bring awareness of the social context into therapy, especially when working with clients who have experienced discrimination, abuse, and domestic and/or systemic violence. In this regard I find narrative practice (White, 2007) a valuable support. Through the process of "externalisation" clients are able to separate the problem from the person, which empowers them to approach the problem from a position of strength rather than that of vulnerability. It can be useful to deconstruct socially induced problems and explore how they function in a person's life. By drawing on the client's unique stories we are able to identify the discourses that shaped their experiences and find ways to challenge them. Overall, narrative practice can effectively be integrated with the Solution Focused approach, as they share a similar postmodernist, social constructivist philosophy ground.

A multidisciplinary approach has become a prominent trend in the understanding of health. The biopsychosocial model (Woods, 2019) of health is widely used by many mental health organisations, including the World Health Organization (WHO). For the practice of Solution Focused therapy, this implies that problems may arise from any of these domains and therefore solutions can be found in any of them, too!

The combination of various domains creates a more holistic, collaborative, and empowering approach to therapy that takes into account both the individual's unique experiences and the broader context in which they occur.

People are more important than theories: I think we are bound to encounter situations when the methods in which we believe so faithfully no longer work. At that moment we need to put aside our favourite manuals and stay open-minded to the reality of the person in front of us. We must be honest about the limits of our competence and – if the client is willing to continue the exploration – create anew what doesn't yet exist.

Which female practitioner inspires you and in which way?

Insoo Kim Berg is one of my constant sources of inspiration. Sometimes, especially in more challenging cases, her words often come to mind:

> Where is my tenacity and ability to hang in there like a pit bull with a bone? It is because of the belief in people, that is, this absolute belief in people that if they have survived this far in their lives, they surely know how to go a little further. Most clients have abilities but they do not believe they do. Therefore, if you do not see it, it is easy to become discouraged (Berg, n.d.).

I recall the women who helped me during my career change. It was a difficult time of transition from manager to psychologist, which gave rise to many doubts and impostor syndrome. My friends supported me, some with words, others with practical advice or even through an opportunity to try out new things, and somehow they all expressed their complete confidence that I would succeed.

It made me think: How did they manage to do it? What was so special in their support that I believed them before proving it?

I want to share a meaningful personal story. In 2011 I translated a workshop for narrative practitioners Sarah Walther and Amanda Redstone. After the workshop I had a correspondence with Sarah asking if she thought I could become a psychologist. She responded in an empowering way encouraging me to pursue my dream and shared her belief that I would become an amazing therapist. She wrote that in the similar way as I was able to create a calm listening space for the workshop participants, I would be able to offer warm and acknowledging space to people in distress. I remember printing out this letter and keeping it in a folder next to my case notes. It really warmed my heart and supported me throughout the years.

I suppose that what Sarah did is a special skill of many women: to see a person in an appreciative and truthful way. Solution Focused therapist Yvonne Dolan calls it "evidence-based compliments"; a compliment that is not praise, which may be of the superficial, "good doggy" type, but rather an acknowledgement of something that is already present. This authentic response elicits trust and allows the person to feel really "seen" – and through another's eyes to recognise their own worth and build on this to step into the future.

What soft small notion would you encourage other women practitioners to embrace?

I would like to share the notion of "Solution Focused embrace".

I find the idea that our pain and suffering can reveal our deepest values very supportive. As Leonard Cohen sang, "There is a crack, a crack in everything // that's how the light gets in". The distress we feel is our response to what happens to us. By embracing it we can discover the things we hold dear and embrace those.

This practice starts before even asking any questions. First, take the time to ground yourself and place your focus within your body. This might involve taking a few deep breaths, stretching, or simply focusing your attention on your physical sensations. You can think of a time when what you did was appreciated, when you were enough as you are. Now direct your attention to the space around you. Imagine yourself in a space where there is room for everything, including that "crack", the problem the client brings or your difficulties in the therapeutic process. Imagine that this space is more than enough, both for you and the client, that it is so vast that it can contain both the presenting problem and the preferred future that might unfold.

By being accepting towards ourselves we can help our clients learn to be accepting towards themselves; and together, to overcome what is impossible alone.

My best hopes for other female Solution Focused voices

Больше всего я надеюсь, что появится больше женщин, практикующих ориентированный на решение подход, и они смогут привнести в работу свои уникальные качества, знания и опыт. Выход терапии за рамки индивидуальной вербальной терапии, большее осознание связи тела-сознания и влияния социального контекста может давать людям ощущение опоры и связи с более широкой сетью поддержки. Я считаю, что именно женщины могут взять на себя ведущую роль в превращении мира в более дружелюбного места для жизни.

My best hope is that there are more female Solution Focused practitioners who can contribute their unique qualities and skills, and help create recognition of the value of feminine qualities in our society and therapeutic work. Expanding our practice beyond individual talk therapy to include bodymind and community awareness can empower clients and give them a sense of belonging to a wider support net. I believe women can take the lead in making the world a more supportive place.

Author reflection

This reflection allowed me to trace the influence of the women who helped me to become who I am, and the unique qualities and strengths they possess, and to better connect to the important people in my life and the values we share.

It was challenging to translate my own implicit female experiences into an explicit form. There is a good Solution Focused question: "How do you manage to do it?" I asked myself this question throughout the writing process, and it helped me delve deeper. Now, having done that, I am more confident that my emphasis on co-presence and support is vital, both for my own path as a trainer and in my role as a supervisor in other, traditionally more masculine, protocol-based approaches.

Co-constructive editors' reflections

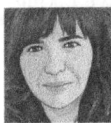

Anne-Marie, I love this chapter. Olga is an amazing woman. There are lots of things that stand out for me about her chapter, but something that I really related to is that her Solution Focused journey started with her motherhood. And it happened to me as well. I really related to how she wrote that becoming a mother and becoming Solution Focused kind of happened at the same time. I felt as though somebody had gone on a similar journey to mine and I really connected to her. And she talks about her belief in people's resilience and how it is all about hope and resilience, and this really resonated with me.

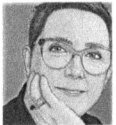

Yes, it's just beautiful. I've put little hearts all over it because I really just love some of her ways of expressing things. Olga is very conscious about the idea of gender, you know, and it was refreshingly different from some other chapters. There are differences, and I have noticed that qualities and activities traditionally considered feminine tend to be neglected and even marginalised. It's about the inner life, and Olga talks about how women should take the lead in their own lives, and I get the feeling that she does, she takes the lead in her life. She says that she is here to help women, to empower women to take the lead. And it is very clear in her chapter that she thinks women should use their intuition.

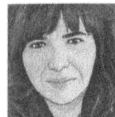

For me, the one thing that stood out in her chapter was this whole idea that we shouldn't lose emotion and intuition in favour of technique and action. Exactly right. And this whole idea that we use a technique at the expense of empathy and our own intuition as women, our authentic self. And she says we need to promote the exchange of implicit knowledge and that intuition is implicit knowledge we all have.

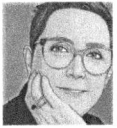

There is also a sense of a strong female perspective. A strong female voice, in a very gentle way. When Olga talks about other theories such as narrative therapy, and the landscape of identity, it is in a way a metaphor, and I could actually use that in a Solution Focused conversation and still be Solution Focused. This reminded me about ideas on the Solution Focused approach as a meta-theory. And maybe that is what Olga's doing, too, because she puts it so beautifully: "My work is based on collaboration".

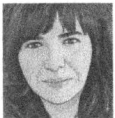

So, the methods and techniques are selected according to the client's preferences and the task at hand. The Solution Focused approach is like a meta-theory and she will tailor-make the therapy, using, adapting, and adding her ideas from other approaches to suit the client. I think it talks about flexibility and matching techniques to suit the client. I like the way it's fluid and interweaving.

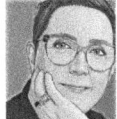

Yes, and it is as if she is saying that for her it is a process of becoming and being not just a technique.

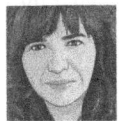

She also talks about this multidisciplinary approach, a biopsychosocial model that embeds the whole human.

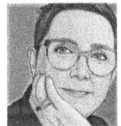

And that makes perfect sense to me. If we take a more holistic view, we see the whole person. Of course, it can also be on a biopsychosocial level. I love looking at people in that way, which reminds me of being eclectic and talking about emotions, that we have the opportunity to talk about them, which many of our contributors refer to and integrate into Solution Focused conversations.

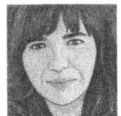

And I mean, that is another, you call it a red thread, I call it a golden thread that comes through. Go to emotions, work with the emotions, use your own emotions, and bring emotions into the approach. Olga also talks about embodiment and non-verbal language, which are actually not mentioned that often in the Solution Focused world, and I think it is necessary to add it to our work.

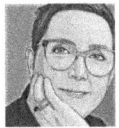

Yes, body language, we don't talk about it. And I love how she watches a client's body language and uses that as a clue or hint to when to ask a question.

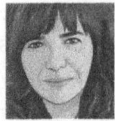

Exactly, and I mean, that is such a shortcut to impact and brevity because she watches their non-verbal body language and uses it as a subtle change and then asks a question. Just brilliant.

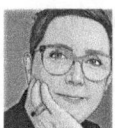

She makes it sound so easy. When you look at microanalysis and the work that Janet Bavelas did with others, they looked at all of Steve's or Insoo's videos and at the face-to-face dialogue. Because of my research in microanalysis of text messages, I have often thought that we can see something in face-to-face dialogues that we cannot see when we have the written words. We see facial expressions and observe the formulations, the anchoring, the acceptance, the recognition, and so on. And that is all non-verbal language.

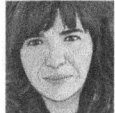

Yes. There's a huge amount that is actually accepted within the Solution Focused world that focuses on non-verbal language that nobody has written about. And I got so excited about this because Olga is saying to all of us out there, we're not writing about this enough, and we're missing a very important part. I got so excited because she's talking about moving to solution land, and she's doing it with more than words. She's using the whole person to help them become what they want because it's a process of becoming. She's not just using words … We're missing a shortcut.

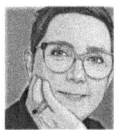

I like the idea of a shortcut, and want to link it back to another thing I loved – when Olga said that we shouldn't use technology at the expense of empathy for people, as it is more important than theory. What really interested me was when she said, "I think we are bound to encounter situations when the methods in which we believe so faithfully no longer work". I've wondered for a long time, how do we know that the method no longer works? We only have the client to tell us. For me, it's not about whether the method works or not; it's about whether it's helpful for the client. We need to constantly check back with the client. It's not about therapists believing faithfully in a method, because if you don't think the Solution Focused approach works, well, it won't. You have to trust the model. It's about checking with the client, "How useful is the way I work for you?" And this is connected to the fact that Olga constantly tailors the sessions and therapy to suit the client. And I love when she says that we have to be brave and we have to create new things that don't exist in order to be innovative, which I actually think Solution Focused ideas allow us to be. And that is also why Olga can write this beautiful chapter, where she talks about the story and an embodiment angle, taking a little of one and a little of the other, all to be most useful to the client.

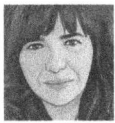

And I kind of feel Olga is saying, I'm not going to apologise for integrating and being flexible. But in actual fact, she's saying we need to be more flexible because the client comes first. And what the client needs, we need to adapt to.

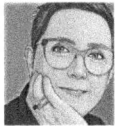

So, it's in a way meaningless to talk about being a purist, because that doesn't say anything about what you do and what you don't do, and how you do it in interaction with others. I was once told by Harry Korman that the Solution Focused approach is about what is "in between the noses". It's not between the ears, it's not inside or outside in the system; it's in between the noses of people to be observed. I love that metaphor.

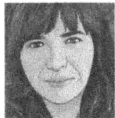

And Olga is suggesting that not only do we have to watch other people's body language and non-verbals but we also have to ground ourselves and our body. We need to ground ourselves physically in order to embrace what is in between the noses.

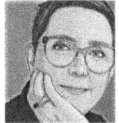

And it made me think maybe we should become aware of our non-verbal communication and our small bodily shifts as the client is talking, as that is a clue to the cracks, because she talks about looking through the cracks.

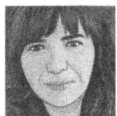

I love the exercises, one that you need to do and one that you need to imagine; actively using an activity to bring the body back into the session, incorporating all of the person. This is a very holistic view of the person, which I really, really like. And it made me think, when she said, Solution Focused embrace, if you think in English about the word embrace, if you embrace somebody, you're hugging them, right? It's a hug. Olga kind of makes me think that what we are doing is hugging the person.

Author references

Berg, I.K. (n.d.). *Hot tips*. South Dakota State University. https://www.sdstate.edu/sites/defa ult/files/2018-06/hot_tips.pdf

Duncan, B.L., Miller, S.D., Wampold, B.E., & Hubble, M.A. (2010). *Heart & soul of change: Delivering what works in therapy*. American Psychological Association.

Henden, J. (2014, 22 March). *"Working with trauma and stress in SFBT"* [Materials]. Workshop, Moscow.

Palmer, W., & Crawford, J. (2013). *Leadership embodiment: How the way we sit and stand can change the way we think and speak*. CreateSpace Independent Publishing Platform.

Rakhmanova, A. (2010). *BabyContact groups for mothers and babies: A psychologist's view*. http://babycontact.ru/about/article/article_babycontact_psychologists_view/ [In Russian]

Rogers, C.R. (1995). *Way of being*. Houghton Mifflin.

White, M. (2007). *Maps of narrative practice*. WW Norton.

Woods, S.B. (2019). Biopsychosocial theories. In B.H. Fiese, M. Celano, K. Deater-Deckard, E.N. Jouriles & M.A. Whisman (Eds.), *APA handbook of contemporary family psychology: Foundations, methods, and contemporary issues across the lifespan* (pp. 75–92). American Psychological Association.

Editor references

De Jong, P., Bavelas, J. B., & Kormann, H. (2013). An introduction to using microanalysis to observe co-construction in psychotherapy. *Journal of Systemic Therapies*, *32*(3), s. 17–30.

McKergow, M., & Korman, H. (2008). *Inbetween: Not inside, nor outside*. Norwegian Agency for Shared Services in Education and Research. https://www.sikt.nu/wp-content/uploads/2015/06/Inbetween-Mark-McKergow-and-Harry-Korman-2008.pdf

Chapter 12

Everyone can benefit from Solution Focused ideas

Kids' Skills training in China

Hongyan Li (China)

Introduction

I worked in the telecommunications industry for 30 years and entered the Solution Focused field at the age of 50. I live in Finland and often go to China, as my daughter studies there. While in China I realised that parents, children, and schools were in dire need of support and connection. Here I found my passion and purpose – in training women, children, and schools in the Kids' Skills approach.

Reflect on how your gender influences your work–life and being a Solution Focused practitioner

Various studies indicate that women are in many ways more sensitive than their male counterparts. They have more empathy and are better at social interaction and emotional processing. I crossed over to the Solution Focused coaching field quite late. As a Solution Focused practitioner, I feel that my gender, sensitivity, empathy, and age have become strengths that help me build rapport with my clients more easily. All the challenges that I previously encountered have become the resources that help me understand and support my clients more effectively.

I believe in the unique strength of women, combining resilience and gentleness, which aligns perfectly with Solution Focused thinking. In *Dao De Jing*, a Chinese philosophical text by Lao Tzu from the sixth century BC，there is a saying, "The highest good is like water", which emphasises the virtue and power of remaining calm, gentle, selfless, and flexible like water. Being a Solution Focused practitioner keeps me humble and inspires me to grow. It means embarking on an endless path of spiritual cultivation.

What is your good reason for staying a Solution Focused practitioner?

I worked in the telecommunications field for 30 years. I moved to Finland with my family when our daughter was three years old and later returned to Beijing to work when our daughter entered college. After working and living in Finland for

DOI: 10.4324/9781003430254-13

17 years, returning to my home country was a huge culture shock. An ongoing company merger, the impact of a new position in the company, and a whole new working environment, as well as conflicts between my personal goals and job requirements, presented me with many challenges and even confusion. To overcome this, in 2010–2011 I spent most of my spare time participating in an extensive Solution Focused coaching programme. I found that Solution Focused coaching resonated with me; the Solution Focused questions woke me up. I was fascinated and tried it with two female friends who felt a desperate need to make changes in their lives. The outcome was a great surprise and inspiration to me. I was amazed at the power of Solution Focused coaching and realised that helping others gives me joy and meaning. My trainer, Dr Marilyn W. Atkinson, told us that, as a coach, you need to figure out your own "niche", the group of people you care about the most. What was my niche? I decided to pursue my passion wholeheartedly by resigning from my job.

When I returned to Beijing in 2008, I saw significant changes had taken place in China while I had been abroad. Fierce competition was everywhere, even in the education field. Everyone was discussing the importance of "not letting children lose at the starting point". It's quite common for parents to enrol their children in diverse tutoring classes at an early age. This trend leads to increased anxiety in parents, exhausted teachers, and unhappy children. The relationship between parents and children, as well as parents and schools, had become tense, and it was not uncommon for young children to suffer from depression. I experienced a strong desire to support Chinese parents and their children, and to help parents discover the joy of raising their children.

I have always admired Finland's child-centred educational philosophy. I believe that Chinese educators and parents can benefit from learning about Finnish education, but wondered how this could happen.

The Bible teaches: "Ask and it will be given to you; seek and you will find; knock and the door will be opened to you". And, sure enough, I encountered Kids' Skills, which is an internationally recognised Solution Focused method for helping children overcome difficulties and problems by learning skills with the support of their family and friends. The ideas of Kids' Skills are 100% in concert with Finland's child-centred educational philosophy. One of the founders of the method is Dr Ben Furman, a psychiatrist, psychotherapist, and internationally renowned expert on Solution Focused psychology, who lives in Helsinki not far from my home. My first meeting with Dr Furman was memorable and I found my calling at that moment.

Kids' Skills is a wonderful step-by-step method. I fell in love with it at first sight and was so thrilled that I wanted to try it immediately. My very first case was working with an 11-year-old boy and his family whom I had met at a school. The school was located on the outskirts of Beijing and was sponsored by private donations and charitable foundations. Many of the children in that school were from poor and disadvantaged families who had moved to Beijing to find work. The boy's parents were working class and had limited time to spend with their son. They didn't know how to deal with the boy's problems other than hitting and scolding him. So, the boy developed a strong tendency towards violence and frequently fought with other children at school and in his neighbourhood. His mother explained that he had recently begun to resist parental discipline with violence. "I don't know what to do. I think he will kill us sooner or later", she said. I started a conversation with the boy and his mother using Kids' Skills. "So, what skill would you like your son to learn?" After discussing it with the mother and the boy, the boy agreed to learn the skill of "having good manners" and named the skill "dignity". Obviously, he cared about his dignity and understood that "having good manners" would bring him dignity. He decided to practise this skill every day at home with his parents in two ways: first, by saying "Goodbye" to his parents when he was leaving for school in the morning, and second, by replying kindly to his mother when she asked him to come to dinner when he was playing games. "Yes, Mom, I am coming", he was supposed to say. He invited his parents to be his supporters and planned the celebration for mastering the skill. He also picked an idol, a popular Chinese singer, as his imaginary supporter. He hoped that one day he would become a respected person like his idol. I promised to send him a signed photo of the singer for his celebration. During several follow-up sessions, I witnessed the boy changing significantly. What surprised me most was the changes in his parents, who learned to appreciate their son and support him in a healthier way. The mother was very grateful and said that Kids' Skills brought laughter back to their family and changed the atmosphere at home. She was also proud of her son because their neighbours had noticed the boy's transformation and had said something along the lines of, "What happened to your son?" One neighbour even visited their home hoping to find out about their parenting secrets. The parents changed dramatically, along with their son. The change in this family proved to me that most parents want to be good parents; they just need to learn some parenting skills.

During this school visit, I also helped a few other children with different problems. These experiences gave me great encouragement and joy. I knew that I had made the right decision.

Helping others is helping oneself. Harvard University Prof. Tal Ben-Shahar said in his famous lecture about happiness,

> Happiness is not a fixed quantity, where if you have more, I must have less. Instead, it can be contagious. One candle can light a thousand candles, and the candle does not burn out any faster. The same is true for sharing happiness, sharing it does not make it diminish (Ben-Shahar, n.d.).

To me, being a Solution Focused practitioner and spreading ideas such as Kids' Skills to reach more people is to share my happiness and to infect more people. In turn, it changes my inner world and my life.

What would others notice you doing that would tell them that you work from a Solution Focused approach?

Over the years, I have translated many important works by Dr Furman into Chinese and introduced him to China, where he has been teaching Solution Focused methods, including Kids' Skills and "Reteaming", since 2013. We have organised dozens of Solution Focused workshops or seminars for Chinese people given by Dr Furman in the past ten years.

We also established the "Kids' Skills Promotion Center" in Beijing in 2014. With the support of Dr Furman, a team of coaches was established to spread Kids' Skills in the country. So far, we have 75 certified Kids' Skills ambassadors and 27 certified facilitators of "Kids' Skills for Parents" who work in their own cities.

Currently, some online programmes are available to allow people to join our learning community at any time, including:

- "Joyful parenting for new Kids' Skills learners" – targeted at ordinary parents and anyone who is interested in Kids' Skills.
- "Growth camp for Kids' Skills teachers" – targeted at elementary school teachers who wish to learn to apply Kids' Skills with the entire class.
- "Solution Focused Brief Therapy, an in-depth online course with Ben Furman" – targeted at Solution Focused coaches.

My aspiration is to make Solution Focused concepts accessible to all parents, caregivers, and teachers through Kids' Skills training. Leveraging the power of the Internet, we can now reach people in all corners of China. Recognising that teachers hold significant sway over both children and parents, we are prioritising efforts to educate and support this group.

The programme "Growth camp for Kids' Skills teachers" is founded on the "Skilful Class" project designed by Dr Furman, the aim of which is to help primary school teachers improve classroom atmosphere, pupils' teamwork skills, school performance, and the general well-being of the children. We hope to build a platform where Chinese school teachers who are interested in Kids' Skills can meet online, learn to use the method, grow together, and empower one another. This programme also involves several Solution Focused games. The teacher can facilitate these games in the class to improve relationships, warm up the atmosphere, and give the students a taste of joyful learning. The pupils are encouraged to take such games home and play them with their families, thereby engaging their parents.

Although our target group of "Growth camp for Kids' Skills teachers" consists of primary school teachers, quite often parents and Kids' Skills coaches join in because they are interested in introducing the project to the schools their children attend. Many teachers stay with us for years and become great examples for newcomers. With this programme, we offer the Kids' Skills coaches a chance to work with local teachers as supporters. We also invite the teachers to share their practising stories regularly through interactive live streaming to further promote Kids' Skills to the public, and so engage even more teachers and parents.

Through these ongoing seminars, workshops, and programmes, we are spreading Solution Focused ideas to everyday people in China. Our Kids' Skills coaches actively support a range of Solution Focused learning groups and educators, from schools to kindergartens, helping to apply Kids' Skills in their communities. As a result, more and more parents and teachers are benefiting from this powerful approach.

Share an exercise that might be useful to other women practitioners

The Circle technique is an interviewing tool developed by Ben Furman and Arnoud Huibers (2022), a psychologist and psychotherapist from the Netherlands. It's a very simple, enjoyable yet effective way to start a coaching session. Whether you coach adults, children, couples, or even a team, the Circle technique can quickly help you build rapport with your client, discover their strengths, talents, abilities, resources, and goals, while making them feel better about themselves and creating a suitable atmosphere for the conversation. In addition, the knowledge and information obtained through the Circle technique help to build solutions together with your clients as the conversation continues.

With the consent of the client, you draw two circles on a sheet of paper, an inner circle and an outer one. You make the inner circle large, asking the client about their strengths, talents, resources, and progress, writing down the information in the inner circle using keywords. Then you proceed to the outer circle, asking the client what they want to change or improve and jotting down two or more such goals in the outer circle.

When you now ask your client to choose which one of their goals they want to focus on, the ensuing conversation will almost automatically become Solution Focused.

Share how you adapt the approach and make it your own. Give us five characteristics that are a part of your Solution Focused DNA

Solution Focused thinking has a positive impact on me in many ways. By prioritising "goals and progress" and acknowledging each other's contributions, we cultivate a positive collaborative atmosphere among the team of Kids' Skills coaches in China.

The use of scaling questions has helped me maintain a positive outlook on progress and resources, enabling me to embrace a "learning by doing" mentality. I have more courage to take action.

This approach enhances my adaptability and resilience, prompting me to ask, "What shall I do in this situation? What do I want?", rather than defaulting to negative self-talk or blame.

Adopting the Solution Focused belief that "everyone is okay" enables me to approach clients without judgement, empowering them to take control of their lives. This attitude towards others enhances my listening skills and understanding. Solution Focused thinking has helped me adopt a growth mindset, viewing life as a journey of learning. I find greater contentment in the process of pursuing goals than in their outcomes.

Which female practitioner inspires you and in which way?

I have been inspired by my trainer, Dr Marilyn W. Atkinson, who is the founder of Erickson Coaching International. She designed a coach training programme called "The Art & Science of Coaching" in which I participated in 2010. She said, "Be passionate about your life. We become what we consciously dream about!" As I watched her shimmering presence on the stage, a woman of 67 years, I couldn't help but feel inspired to become someone like her – a person driven by passion, dedicated to empowering and uplifting others for as long as possible.

What soft small notion would you encourage other women practitioners to embrace?

Mother Teresa said: "Not all of us can do great things, but we can all do small things with great love". A small step is greater than a giant leap; never underestimate the power of water.

My best hopes for other female Solution Focused voices

中国的KS教练们喜欢说"做行走的KS！"。

做为女性焦点解决践行者，我们是母亲，祖母，女儿，妻子，老师，我们每天都在用自己的言行影响着孩子、家庭和周遭的世界。我们的影响力超出我们的想象。践行SF的理念，可以让我们活出最美的样子，温柔而坚定，共同创建更加和谐平等的社会。

The Kids' Skills coaches in China have a slogan: "Be a walking Kids' Skill!" As female Solution Focused practitioners, we are mothers, grandmothers, daughters, wives, and teachers utilising our words and actions to influence our children, families, and people around us in our everyday lives. The impact we make on the world is beyond our imagination. By practising Solution Focused principles, we live out our best selves and demonstrate gentleness and firmness when we work to create a more harmonious and equitable society.

Author's reflection

Everyone can benefit from Solution Focused thinking, regardless of gender or age. As female Solution Focused practitioners, we possess unique advantages in helping our clients while continuously enhancing our abilities. As a central figure in a family, a woman who incorporates Solution Focused principles into her life can create a more heartwarming living experience.

Kids' Skills is a Solution Focused programme designed to help children overcome various challenges and cultivate positive behaviour, making it particularly valuable in schools and kindergartens. This step-by-step approach can help teachers work more effectively while experiencing a sense of reward. Introducing the "Skillful Class" project in primary schools has the potential to foster a more constructive and supportive learning environment for children.

It is essential to form a learning community when promoting Solution Focused ideas such as the Kids' Skills programme. We need to offer a platform for individuals to learn together, exchange their experiences, and empower one another. One person can walk fast, but it takes a group of people to go far. When the right people come together to do the right thing, not only can they go far but they can also spread happiness along the way.

Co-constructive editors' reflection

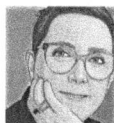 I read Julia's (as Li is known here in Denmark) answer to the first question and was blown away. Wow, all the challenges I've encountered in the past have become the resources that "help me understand and support my clients more effectively". And you get the feeling that it is not only the clients she has supported but also herself on her journey towards becoming a Solution Focused coach. I was truly impressed by the challenges that she so easily transforms into her resources.

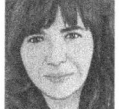 Absolutely, and how she then uses this to build a rapport with the client. And then I was so blown away by her words on combining resilience and gentleness. The metaphor of water and how it is calm, gentle, selfless, and flexible, how it keeps her humble and is the path of spiritual cultivation. I don't know why, but I never thought of resilience being gentle. I love her passion for helping families in China. She calls it a niche, but it is clear that this way of working helps her to help people find joy in parenting and raising their children.

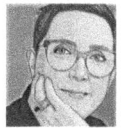 I was also struck by her descriptions about developments in China in the parenting role, and the shift in the importance of not letting children "lose at the starting point". It sounds harsh and as though they need to perform all the time. Julia has this passion for improving the relationship between children and parents.

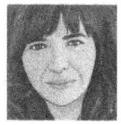 And I love that she said that Solution Focused questions woke her up. It's like the approach woke her up to say, here is something that works, something that I can use within my context.

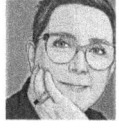 And I think this is exactly what she is doing. Help parents and children discover joy again. Which makes me think how wonderful it is that she is focusing on the interactive perspective between parents and children.

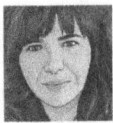

And a little bit later, she also says it brings "laughter back into the home". The laughter and appreciation for each other makes them feel proud of each other again. I'll never forget Ben Furman saying at a workshop that we have to create praise instead of panic. And she brings praise and pride and appreciation back into the family context.

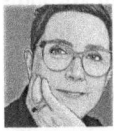

Yes, and further on, "it changes my inner world and my life". I was really moved by this.

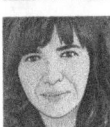

And then she says, she can reach more people and "infect" people. It's not "affect" people, she can infect others. It's like this joy, happiness, and laughter can, like a virus, be infected back into people. And that changes her inner world. Her Solution Focused virus is that she wants to infect every ordinary person, every ordinary parent who wants to learn with joy, appreciation, and happiness.

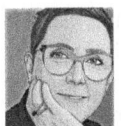

And there's a huge population in China and a lot of work to be done. Julia and Ben are ambitious and focused, reaching so many people on so many levels. It's quite impressive, the work she has established along with Ben.

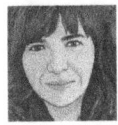

I love that Julia is reminding us how accessible the Solution Focused approach is, using it with children, parents, and teachers, as well as coaches, teams, couples, and nearly anybody else who wants to learn.

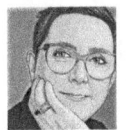

And then thinking of the presuppositions that have an impact on her and her being. She really believes that you can be in a not-knowing position and that the client is the expert of their own life. This belief enables her to "approach clients without judgement, empowering them to take control of their lives".

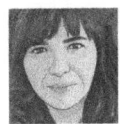

Absolutely. And that they can take control of their own lives, which shows that she assumes, from the word go, that everyone is capable and that everyone is okay. And for that reason she focuses on progress and scaling progress. Almost as though she is saying, "Okay, so let's move forward, let's look at pursuing goals and progress".

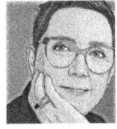

Julia reminds us that there is a great satisfaction in the process towards the goal, and not only in reaching the result. Steve de Shazer talked about goals versus solutions and the impact of achieving the goal. The solution is the effect or result of achieving the goal, so if the goal is, "I want to get an education", then the effect is 1) I can get a job, 2) I can earn my own money, 3) I can buy a house, 4) I can buy a car, and so on. It is the result or solution to achieve that goal. However, Julia talks about the process of achieving the goal.

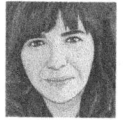

Yes, what Julia is saying is that the journey of reaching the goal, that process is just as valuable and just as important as the outcome. And in her case, she thinks that the journey of reaching or finding the goal or pursuing it is most valuable. It makes me think of the first Steve de Shazer workshop I ever attended. I wrote in my notes and on my handout: "Slow down, Jacqui". And what Julia has reminded me of is enjoying the journey. Slow down, enjoy the journey. Look around. Look at what you see before you come to that end destination. Because there are beautiful sights and scenes along the way.

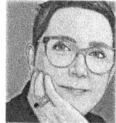

Yes, and for me, it's "Whenever you want to go fast, go slow". That really helps me to step back. I think she's right: we need to pay attention to the process.

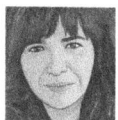

Yes, and then she ends her chapter again by reminding us that "small things with great love" can make such a big impact. The whole idea of doing it with "a heart of love" is beautiful … You might think it's a small thing, but it can make such a big impact and create such great change. And again, she reminds us that we live our best selves with gentleness and firmness. I love that.

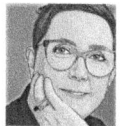

Yes, Julia has a philosophy, in a sense, where the Solution Focused approach fits into her ideas and her beliefs. I get the impression when she quotes Mother Teresa that not all of us can do great things, but we can do small things with great love, that she is doing this with so much love. Love for China, love for children, love for making a difference. And also love and hope for affecting the beliefs of parents about their children and society.

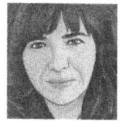

Yes. And with this great, great love she believes that parents can find love and joy with their children again. I agree: we can't all do great things, but we can do small things, and I think with all her small things put together she's doing great things.

Author references

Atkinson, M.W., & Chois, R.T. (2012a). *Step-by-step coaching*. Exalon Publishing.

Atkinson, M.W., & Chois, R.T. (2012b). *Flow: The core of coaching*. Exalon Publishing.

Ben-Shahar, T. (n.d.). *Positive psychology: The science of happiness*. [Video]. YouTube. https://www.youtube.com/watch?app=desktop&v=wBWejfL0xOA&t=5640s

Ben-Shahar, T. (2007). *Happier: Learn the secrets to daily joy and lasting fulfilment*. McGraw Hill.

Berg, I.K., & de Jong, P. (2007). *Interviewing for solutions* (4th ed.). Cengage Learning.

Furman, B. (1998). *Never too late to have a happy childhood: From adversity to resilience*. BT Press.

Furman, B. (2004). *Kids' Skills: Playful and practical Solution-Finding with children.* St Luke's Innovative Resources.

Furman, B., & Ahola, T. (1992). *Solution talk: Hosting therapeutic conversations.* W.W. Norton.

Furman, B., & Ahola, T. (2007). *Changing through cooperation: Handbook of reteaming.* Lyhytterapia-instituutti.

Furman, B., & Huibers, A. (2022). The Solution-Focused Circle technique: A visual tool for discovering strengths and facilitating change in therapy and counseling. *Journal of Solution Focused Practices, 6*(2). https://doi.org/10.59874/001c.75018

Lao Zi (2021). *Dao De Jing.* ZHBC.

Editor reference

De Shazer, S. (n.d.). *Goals & solutions: A useful distinction.* Norwegian Agency for Shared Services in Education and Research. https://www.sikt.nu/wp-content/uploads/2020/11/goals-solutions.pdf

Chapter 13

Solution Focused supervision from the perspective of gender and culture

Jane Tuomola (Singapore)

Introduction

After many years of working in the UK, I moved to Singapore in 2008 and trained in the Solution Focused approach in 2009. I have my own private practice here working as a clinical psychologist and coach. My clients are a mix of Singaporeans and expatriates from around the globe. I have done supervision for over 15 years, and supervise individuals and groups of mental health professionals in Singapore hospitals, schools, and non-profit organisations. I also work as a trainer, supervisor, and mentor coach with the Academy of Solution Focused Training in Asia and SolutionsAcademy in Europe. There is a wonderful community of Solution Focused practitioners in Singapore who regularly meet and support each other. There is also a global online community where I can ask questions or discuss ideas with top people in the field. In this chapter I share my thoughts about supervision from the perspective of gender and culture.

Reflect on how your gender influences your work–life and being a Solution Focused practitioner

I grew up in a family that valued education and serving others. I went to an all-girls secondary school and was encouraged to work hard and achieve. My mum always worked and, while she changed her career to be a teacher after having children and so be available during the holidays, it is something she was good at and enjoyed. I therefore never saw my gender as an obstacle.

I am now a busy working mum of two children. Both my children and my work are important, so I am often juggling multiple roles and end up putting my own needs last. There is never enough time in the day to do all I would like. I feel being a working mum is about constantly making choices, having a heavy mental load, and feeling guilty that some part of my life is suffering. I feel both lucky that I get to make these choices and at times also resent having to do so.

In my work life this has led me to focus on supporting other women managing similar transitions. I can empathise with the challenges they face and love helping other women who are juggling multiple demands to clarify what they want and

DOI: 10.4324/9781003430254-14

what the right balance is for them. The Solution Focused approach is a wonderful way of doing this, as I can explore what each client wants that fits their hopes and desires and cultural context.

What is your good reason for staying a Solution Focused practitioner?
The simple answer is that it works. As a clinical psychologist who used to teach evidence-based practice, it is important to me to use a model that is effective.

There are many approaches with a solid research evidence base, though, so the reason I choose the Solution Focused approach is because it is the most respectful of and empowering to clients. Asking questions about clients' successes helps them connect with their strong, resourceful side instead of with the hopeless and over-whelmed person who had walked through my door. I learn from and am inspired by the creativity and brilliance of my clients as much as they do and are. A Solution Focused conversation is empowering, as it turns what can seem an insurmountable challenge into manageable steps forward. By being client led rather than expert driven, it honours the goals the client wants to achieve. The preferred future is set by the client from their frame of reference, so it works well across different cultural contexts, for example, and with a diverse range of clients.

An exercise I do when training others in the Solution Focused approach is comparing problem-focused versus Solution Focused interviewing. I am always stunned that in only five minutes the difference is obvious. I would much rather work in a way that leaves both the therapist and the client feeling hopeful and ener-gised rather than overwhelmed and demoralised.

In terms of supervision, a quote from Insoo Kim Berg summarises the import-ance to me of taking a Solution Focused approach in supervision:

> This new posture (SF) reduces the defensiveness of those being managed or supervised, thus staff rise to the challenge and start to think for themselves and taking actions based on this sense of competence, rather than always defending his/her position. Not allowing supervisees ... to lower themselves to a defensive position is the most respectful, empowering and yet demanding posture we can take (Berg, n.d).

What would others notice you doing that would tell them that you work from a Solution Focused approach?

Being Solution Focused is about being collaborative and co-constructing in both the content and process of conversations. I start supervision sessions exploring best hopes *from* the session and best hopes *for* the session, i.e., how we would need to be together to enable their best hopes to happen. This is different to supervisees' previous experiences, where the supervisor leads as the expert.

Conversations using a Solution Focused approach focus on the desired future (rather than explanations of the problematic past) and on the successful past (what is already working rather than what is not). During supervision, I ask questions that help supervisees to describe their preferred future in relation to a specific topic or client issue. I ask what ideas they have already had, what they have done that has worked well in similar situations that they could apply here, and how they would notice moving one small step forwards from where they are to where they want to be.

Having used the Solution Focused approach for so long that it has become how I see the world and other people, it is sometimes hard to remember how unusual this is for mental health professionals trained in problem-focused approaches. One counsellor (private communication) shared the following, which sums up the approach perfectly:

> I liked the questions. After the session I left with a sense of clarity and a multitude of ideas regarding what I could do with the client. Rather than feeling demoralised and overwhelmed, I felt affirmed by the supervision process, as the questions asked centred on my strengths.

Share an exercise that might be useful to other women practitioners

Therapists care deeply about making a difference in clients' lives. Yet working in the field of mental health is challenging, and having a safe space to reflect on your work is invaluable. Most supervisees bring only challenging cases where they are stuck. While an important part of supervision, this can easily take up all the time and take the focus away from the therapist and their own growth.

I ask all supervisees to complete this exercise adapted from Dolan (1998, p. 66) and Freeman (2011). This allows the supervisee to focus on hopes for themselves and helps us co-create the supervision process. It can be used with individual supervisees or in a group (where common themes relevant to everyone are identified). It can also be done alone and taken to your own supervisor.

Supervision email from the future

Pick a point in time 6–24 months from now. Send me an email from this future time as though you are looking back at the positive changes that have happened in your practice as a therapist.

Include a description of your typical work week (in the present tense). Describe in detail what you are pleased to notice about your work as a therapist. What are you pleased that you have been maintaining over time? What is better, new, or different now compared to when we first started supervision that shows you have grown as a therapist during this time? Now that these changes have happened in your work – what do you notice about your life outside work? In what ways is this future a good place to be? Who else will notice these changes? What will they notice?

In what ways was supervision helpful to you in making these changes and what key factors came from your part and what came from mine?

Share how you adapt the approach and make it your own. Give us five characteristics that are a part of your Solution Focused DNA

Leading from one step behind: the supervisee and supervisor relationship is inherently unequal and hierarchical. As a supervisor, I have a duty to uphold the ethical principles of my profession and protect clients while supporting the supervisee's learning. Training as a Solution Focused practitioner has helped flatten this hierarchy. I identify with the idea of leading from one step behind (Cantwell & Holmes, 1994). Seeing the supervisee as the expert in their own work context, and trusting that they have their own strengths and resources, has meant I now show up in a different way in my supervision sessions. As Pichot and Dolan state: "The role of the Solution Focused supervisor is to pull the wisdom from the therapists rather than tell them what to do" (2003, p. 173). It was, however, also helpful for me to learn that the idea that Solution Focused supervisors do not give direction was a myth and that "[e]ffective supervisors must acquire the ability to determine when they need to provide information and when simply listening to the staff members will be more productive" (Pichot & Dolan, 2003, p. 171).

Complimenting appropriately: by asking about what is working for supervisees, it is easy to reflect these successes through compliments. In the Asian context, where modesty and humility are cultural values, it is important to be mindful of complimenting appropriately. Offering more indirect compliments and doing so in a gentle manner works better than being overly effusive. Being explicit about the purpose of compliments and empathising that I understand it can feel awkward initially is helpful. Over time, supervisees see that receiving compliments prior to suggestions helps them take on board the suggestions from a position of competence rather than that of feeling criticised. This fits well with another important Asian cultural value of not losing face or being shamed in front of others.

Being a scientist practitioner: as a psychologist and scientist practitioner, keeping up with research to help my direct client work and in supervising and training others is important. However, I also stay true to how the Solution Focused approach started and pay close attention to what works for *my* clients in *my* setting in order to combine what the research says at a macro level with practice-based evidence at the micro level. I collected many of these stories in the book *Solution Focused practice in Asia* (Hogan et al., 2017) to help others in the region use Solution Focused ideas in a way that is "same, same but different".

Being mindful of language and aware of power and privilege: the Solution Focused approach is a language-based approach where conversation is co-created. Training in microanalysis helped me be intentional in my language use, to understand the presuppositions and assumptions embedded in the questions I ask and using the clients' words as far as possible.

The Solution Focused approach has, however, been criticised for ignoring issues of gender and power (Dermer et al., 1998), and exploring Solution Focused questions through the lens of gender has helped me be mindful of other messages I may be transmitting unwittingly. Take the following dialogue:

Therapist: What are your best hopes for this session?
Client: I'm feeling stressed and want to be able to deal with things better.
Therapist: So, what would you notice when you are dealing with things better?

The last question is Solution Focused and builds directly on the client's stated best hopes to create their preferred future. However, what if the client is a woman and the stress is dealing with an abusive husband or bullying boss? This question may therefore inadvertently locate the responsibility of change with the woman, rather than acknowledging the issues of power and injustice in the situation.

Doing a risk assessment with all clients to address immediate safety concerns is important. However, beyond that there can be a fine line between supporting a woman to be the best version of herself and making sure not to imply that it is her job to figure out how best to put up with an unjust or abusive situation.

I try to be aware of issues of power and privilege and when a client may be disempowered or marginalised (not just in relation to gender). In my role as supervisor, I help supervisees be more aware of these issues so that they neither ignore them nor jump in to rescue a client, which may disempower them further.

Which female practitioner inspires you and in which way?

The female practitioner who inspires me most is Debbie Hogan. She was the trainer on my "Foundations of Solution Focused Therapy" course in 2009. Over time she has taken several roles on my Solution Focused journey as my trainer, mentor, coach, and supervisor. Now I work as an associate trainer with her, so she is officially my "boss", but in practice she is a very dear colleague and friend.

Initially, I wasn't particularly interested in the Solution Focused approach but needed Continuing Professional Development hours and a colleague recommended Solution Focused training. Being a clinical psychologist, I subscribed to the importance of assessing, diagnosing, and formulating a client's problems. I was the most sceptical person on the course and could not buy into the Solution Focused assumptions. Debbie met me where I was, and at no point tried to convince me to be Solution Focused. She allowed me to explore my good reasons for being sceptical, and stayed curious about what I was discovering through the experiential exercises. This enabled me to risk letting go of my previous expertise and try something new. She didn't just teach the Solution Focused approach but also embodied it with her kindness and humility – giving credit to others and underplaying her role in creating change.

Her encounter with the Solution Focused approach (Hogan, 2009) closely mirrors my own. It is inspiring to read of her journey coming from a healthcare setting steeped in the medical model and a lens of pathology to finding that the Solution Focused approach is hopeful and transformative for clients.

I also admire her for the impact she has had in bringing the Solution Focused approach to so many individuals, groups, and organisations in Asia (Hogan et al., 2017) in a way that both stays true to the Solution Focused approach and acknowledges the differences needed in this cultural context.

What soft small notion would you encourage other women practitioners to embrace?

I would encourage women practitioners to embrace the art of listening in a Solution Focused way, summed up beautifully by the Chinese character tīng (to listen) in Figure 13.1.

The character tīng is made up of several parts:

- Ear: listening and gathering information about what the client has said.
- King: showing respect and listening as though the person in front of you is as important and valued as a king.
- 10 or maximum: giving clients 100% of your attention.
- Eye: noticing what your client may be communicating non-verbally.
- Heart: listening wholeheartedly to feel what the person needs.
- One: by embracing all these ways of listening we can become of one heart.

My best hopes for other female Solution Focused voices

My best hope is that all women practitioners find their own voices and feel safe to express them. I hope that they trust that they know themselves better than anyone else and what is right for them. I hope that they are able to support and inspire others to do the same.

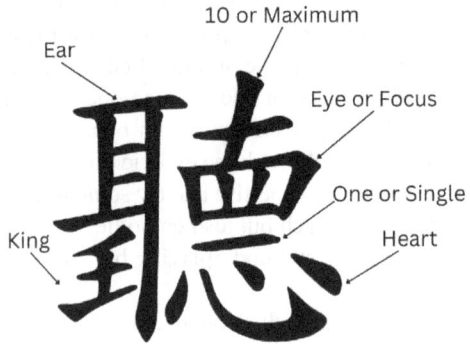

Figure 13.1 "Tīng" – to listen. Illustrated by Cha Chee Seng

Being surrounded by other Solution Focused practitioners who share the same ideas is crucial when living in a problem-focused world. So, my hope is that every practitioner has a wonderful Solution Focused community alongside them in their journey.

Author's reflection

Having lived outside my home country for 15 years, I am used to exploring the impact of cultural context on my work (see Hogan et al., 2017). When asked to contribute to this book, I felt like a fish in the sea unable to see the water in which I was swimming. It has been a useful exercise to consider the impact of gender on my life and work in an explicit way and I am excited to explore this more. I hope my reflections are in some way useful to others and am always happy to connect and be part of your Solution Focused community.

Co-constructive editors' reflections

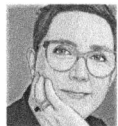 It is interesting to read these background tracks of childhood and how we all mirror our parents, especially our moms. It made me realise the impact of what we are doing to our daughters. When you have enough of these past moments, then you realise, okay, there might be a pattern in this that affects the future and our daughters.

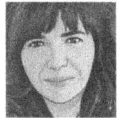 The juggling of motherhood and work life. A constant challenge of making choices, but for Jane this led her to helping other women who have the same difficulties in managing family and work. She calls it transitions. She adds, and this I also can relate to, that she then neglects herself, making these choices where some part of her is suffering.

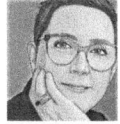 Jane is a professional and she knows exactly what she's doing, and this led to her focusing on helping other women. It's like a motor for her, you know.

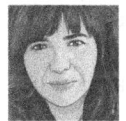 It motivated her, this awareness, to be helpful to other women in similar situations. And I think that's also the big draw card for her, the reason why she is so passionate about supervision.

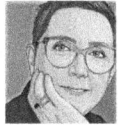 And about coaching, I think Jane wants something evidence-based that is working, and she not only learns from the client's creativity and brilliance, but she also brings forward energy.

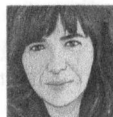

There is a cyclic story in Jane's whole chapter. It's the cycle she goes through with becoming Solution Focused. She was a big sceptic in the beginning as a clinical psychologist, and there was this journey and cycle of getting to a place where she knows it works. And the cycle that she goes through with the client as well, where it goes from overwhelmed and hopeless to creative and brilliant. And she writes later that it becomes the way she sees the world and people. So it has really become her, her whole life philosophy. And what stood out for me about what others would notice is, especially in her role as a supervisor, where often a supervisee comes to you as the expert, how mindful she stays about not being the expert and about relying on the supervisee's creativity and ideas. And she asks her supervisee how they need to be in a session. So she's really including the person who asks for help as a co-expert in the whole process.

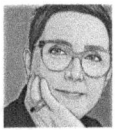

And the exercise is a nice way to get some reflections about standing in the future and looking back, and what makes a difference. I like the questions that go along with this exercise to reflect upon, that is, the whole context, both in your work and in your life outside of work. It goes through the cyclic process of growth and hope.

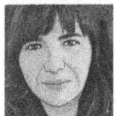

Something that really stood out for me about Jane's chapter is how respectful and mindful she is of the hierarchy. Of complimenting. Respectfully, you know, so that she's constantly aware of not taking a power position and not doing anything that from a cultural place can be disrespectful.

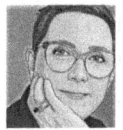

And what really stood out to me was how Jane is acutely aware of the culture she's a part of, a culture that compliments and needs to be appropriate. And it's different when you're in an Asian culture with different values and beliefs. Then you just need to adapt your compliments to the clients in a different and more appropriate way. Yes, I really like that she suggests that we need to be aware of the culture.

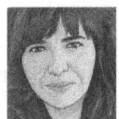

And what I also liked is that she was saying that she is amplifying the obvious strengths of the person, which then empowers them to move towards a place of acceptance and not shame. And I love it. And then how she still stays a researcher. She stays scientific, but always uses Solution Focused principles as her umbrella theory.

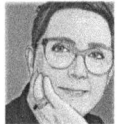

Finally, I noted how Jane is aware of language and aware of power and privilege. This reference to a feminist critique of Solution Focused therapy was new to me, and it was inspiring to read her reflections on this and that the approach has been criticised for ignoring issues of gender and power. Again, she sort of unfolds this and gives us new perspectives on how this could be interpreted.

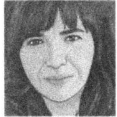 And what Jane consistently does in the chapter is remind us to be mindful, right? To be mindful, respectful, and ethical in a way, to be able to not criticise but rather to evaluate our impact. She included the Chinese character because this is where she works. This is contextually appropriate. And I love how the character's ear, eye, and heart are so Solution Focused. You know, how we listen, how we look, how we observe, and what we believe in people. It's seeing our basic Solution Focused assumptions through a different cultural symbol.

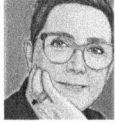 And it's difficult not to welcome and encourage her best hopes; find and feel, for women not only to find but also to feel safe to express their own voices. I love her idea of building a community, a family of Solution Focused people around you on your journey, because she also joined a large welcoming family. So she's encouraging other practitioners to become part of the Solution Focused family.

Author references

Berg, I.K. (n.d.). *Hot tips III: Details, details and more details.* Norwegian Agency for Shared Services in Education and Research. https://www.sikt.nu/wp-content/uploads/2020/11/Insoo_Hot_Tips_ii-v.pdf

Cantwell, P., & Holmes, S. (1994). Social construction: A paradigm shift for systemic therapy and training. *Australia and New Zealand Journal for Family Therapy, 15*(1), 17–26.

Dermer, S.B., Hemesath, C.W., & Russell, C.S. (1998). A feminist critique of Solution-Focused therapy. *American Journal of Family Therapy, 26*(3), 239–250.

Dolan, Y. (1998). *Beyond survival: Living well is the best revenge.* BT Press.

Freeman, S. (2011). Supervision email from the future. In T.S. Nelson (Ed.), *Doing something different: Solution-Focused brief therapy practices.* Routledge.

Hogan, D. (2009). My encounter with the Solution Focused therapy model. In E. Connie & L. Metcalf (Eds), *The art of Solution Focused therapy* (pp. 175–188). Springer Publishing Company.

Hogan, D., Tuomola, J., & Yeo, A. (Eds.) (2017). *Solution Focused practice in Asia.* Routledge.

Pichot, T., & Dolan, Y.M. (2003). Solution Focused supervision: Leading from one step behind. In T. Pichot & Y.M. Dolan (Eds.), *Solution-Focused Brief Therapy: Its effective use in agency settings* (pp. 159–179). The Haworth Press.

Chapter 14

Disruptive thinking
Adventures in Australian veteran support

Jacqui van de Velde (Australia)

Introduction

It was a lovely surprise to be contacted to contribute a chapter to this book. The brilliance of the Solution Focused approach is that it escaped the therapy world and happily infiltrated many disciplines, bringing richness and joy to the work in those fields. The context of this chapter is veteran support in Australia. It is a reflection on how Solution Focused principles are helping to change conversations, focusing and empowering veterans and their families one conversation at a time to live their best lives.

Some of what I do in this sector is volunteer work and some is actual, gainful employment. All of it is potentially a fight. Most of this work really messes with your head and emotions – as well as your understanding and perceptions of justice. Every day I see that what happens to our veterans post-service is far worse than what they are exposed to during service. There is a moral injury that makes matters worse. Veterans describe the actions or inaction of our Department of Veterans Affairs as "delay, deny, wait until we die". Based on what I witness on a daily basis, this is an accurate statement. Australia is currently in the middle of a Royal Commission into Defence and Veteran Suicide (a royal commission is the country's highest form of inquiry into matters of public importance). It is all very raw here at the moment. To say we are in a dark place is an understatement. For those of you who are therapists, imagine an entire caseload and then multiply that out across the country. Also imagine that each time someone pops up to "make a difference", the toxicity of the culture top-down and bottom-up means they are met with scepticism, doubt, and a healthy dose of "We will sit back and watch you fail from here, mate".

DOI: 10.4324/9781003430254-15

Reflect on how your gender influences your work–life and being a Solution Focused practitioner

When I first ventured into a more public role in veteran support, I was warned by well-meaning and trusted friends, "You will fail". I asked why and this is a summary of the responses:

- The powerful influence of large ex-service organisations and their ownership of this space. This "space", as I have come to understand it, is the public square on all matters veteran: policy, politics, social, and community.
- You are not a veteran.
- You are a woman.

There was no malice in their warning. They were simply very good friends expressing the reality of their own experiences. Their warning was also symptomatic of the largely "problem-focused" and "problem-drenched" experiences of veteran support in Australia. Is this surprising? No. Every time an individual or well-meaning group stepped up to help veterans, they would be met with huge barriers. Some of these barriers are the legal and governance requirements, which are arguably good things to have in place. We want good corporate and business citizens. The other barriers are the ones that cause the greatest challenges: white-anting, gaslighting, and hostile business activities, all from other "charitable" organisations supposedly working for the same goals – better life outcomes for our veterans and their families. Reasons? Based on observation, it simply comes down to money and competing for a share of the finite pie of charitable funds and government grants. You can throw a healthy dose of toxic ego into the mix as well. All operating in a legislative framework that is no longer fit for purpose.

I am not a veteran. In many ways not being a veteran actually gives you permission to ask the really tough questions that veterans may be too embarrassed or ashamed to ask or that they, through the circumstances of their service, are prevented from asking.

I am a woman. Reflecting on how being a woman influences my work life is a genuine challenge. For a start, I never refer to my sex. Nor do I consciously view my work life through a gender lens. Early in my professional life I found the feminist movement lacking a certain authenticity. The way the rhetoric morphed into "man-hating" did more to hinder women than it did to promote women as equal partners in all aspects of society. Therefore, it was my conscious decision to counter the experience of toxic feminism. A workplace "sisterhood" is not something I subscribed to. In fact, reflecting on my 30-plus years of professional life, my observation and experience of poor behaviour in the workplace have been of women, towards women. The notion of supporting women purely because they are women has, in my opinion, made women less than their potential and signs individuals up to a class and identity war where nobody wins; it's a distraction. Solution

Focused practices provide a different mindset. Using Solution Focused practices means the politics of sex and gender are no longer relevant.

What is your good reason for staying a Solution Focused practitioner?

My main reason for sticking with the Solution Focused approach is that it gets results. Solution Focused practice promotes authentic relationships. It honours the contribution of each party in a discussion or project. Solution Focused practices have protective factors that remove the barriers created by labelling practices and the trauma-informed approach.

For several years I was on a school board. The school had been established by an Australian Catholic religious order, the Sisters of the Good Samaritan. One of their governance practices for all aspects of their corporate work is the application of the *Regula Sancti Benedicti*, the Rule of St Benedict (AD 530), "Listen with the ear of your heart".[1] I think St Benedict was a Solution Focused practitioner! Even the smallest voice from those perceived as the least important in the hierarchy of monastic life was listened to. St Benedict's Rule gave individuals the permission to express their ideas and solutions. Wisdom and solutions come from the most amazing and sometimes least likely sources. The practice of "listening with the ear of your heart" is quite literally transformational when it comes to engaging with veterans and their families.

Case study 1: A soft landing

I am on the board of the non-profit Wellbeing Australia and the lead for the Veteran Wellbeing Summit (VWS), which started in 2019. VWS is Solution Focused by stealth. We have had some overtly Solution Focused practitioners present and run workshops. The bulk of what we do is gathering people and stories of success in veteran wellbeing and suicide prevention. The focus is on action, hope, and transformation; thus the things that work or are working.

Why is VWS a soft landing? Veterans are a leery bunch. To be honest, if you are living in a culture where to admit injury is failure, where failure is not acceptable, and there is a closely held belief that everything and everyone who is in a supporting position has let you down and will let you down, you are leery. It doesn't matter if this is not universally true; for the veteran coming to a realisation that they need assistance, it is true. VWS gives control back to the participants and allows them to explore solutions in their own space and time; thus a soft landing.

All of our presenters are briefed on the focus and that we are interested in hearing about what is working and how they know it is working, and what evidence there is that it is working. This approach changes the energy in any presentation or discussion. The result is that even when we have presenters dealing with really challenging subject matter, there is always a silver lining. There is a minimum essential kernel of hope that can be gleaned from each presentation.

VWS was online before it became cool and necessary. The big win with this format is that the participant has control; control about what they watch and when they watch – and if they want to participate live, they can. This is where the gamble with presupposition kicks in. In the early planning days I contacted a senior person within the Department of Veterans Affairs seeking some endorsement for what we were planning. The response was not what I was expecting. At worst I thought we would get a "No", at best I was hopeful and thought it would be, "Great idea, how can we support you?" What I got was, "Veterans are vulnerable, we have concerns about them engaging with material that is not trauma informed". Boom! Here was a classic example of the "problem" diversion control mechanism, plus trauma-informed (Fallot & Harris, 2001) labelling. We ignored the "concerns" and presupposed that participants would "opt in", choose the sessions they wanted to view either live or recorded, from home, with the support team they wanted to have with them. It worked.

Data is a wonderful thing! Engagement data: sign-ups, views, clicks, shares; and asking the question, "How useful was this for you?" It has all been far more successful than we could have imagined when we first determined the success criteria. The analysis of what veterans were interested in was affirming and set the course for the next three years:

• Veterans want skills and information so they can manage their own wellbeing, mental and physical health; and
• Partners and families of veterans want the same.

The image of the broken veteran who has wellbeing, mental and physical health "done" to them is not accurate. Solutions and solution talk are popular, as there is no blame, only forward motion. The interactions that held back support in the past are not present when you have democratised access to information and resources in the way we did via a free online summit. There were 16,000 individual views of videos, current and previous, in 2020–2022. The content from VWS might not tick all the Solution Focused boxes for the purists, but it is at its core Solution Focused and it is Solution Focused by stealth.

What would others notice you doing that would tell them that you work from a Solution Focused approach?

I hope that people will notice optimism and hope, clarity and purpose. When I first started with Solution Focused practices, my initial reaction was, "These people are too nice! They are being nice and being walked over." The reality could not be more different. What I misinterpreted as "nice" was actually deep respect and truth. Not relativism or the "your truth, my truth" disingenuous dialogue. But the truth. There is a refreshing revelation of truth in this practice mode.

Share an exercise that might be useful to other women practitioners

The most useful application of Solution Focused practice for me is self-coaching. When you work with other Solution Focused practitioners or have formal supervision as part of your work as a therapist, the coaching is built into the work you do. Working largely on my own and as the only Solution Focused person in the room, I needed to find other ways of reflecting on my practice. As a result I journal, particularly during a project. It is quick and simple, no dark-night-of-the-soul analysis.

- Where am I on the scale of 0–10 today?
- What makes it that number?
- Jot down what worked well and why.
- If it is even better tomorrow, where will I be on the scale and what will have happened, what will I notice, what will I be appreciating?

This should all sound pretty familiar. It keeps my head above water and my eyes on where I want to be and how I want to feel about a project or piece of work.

Share how you adapt the approach and make it your own. Give us five characteristics that are a part of your Solution Focused DNA

When asked to share how I have adapted the Solution Focused approach and made it my own, I can't answer. Truthfully, I am still in a development stage and can't honestly settle on any adaptations, because each conversation and application is different. However, there are lessons that I can share at this point.

Lesson 1: I have come to understand that problem focus is also a method of control. Deploying problems to knock out perceived competition is a real tactic. If we are busy focusing on the problems and in a constant triage mode, we never get to liberate creative thinking to get the solutions we need to implement. The Solution Focused mindset is very simple to apply here. Do not play other people's or organisations' problem games. They are irrelevant and a monumental distraction.

Lesson 2: the Solution Focused approach provides a valuable framework for mindset, negotiating change and empowerment. From a personal perspective and from the perspective of the teams I am working with, IT KEEPS YOU SANE! Solution Focused thinking keeps you focused on what matters in the project. It keeps you focused on the signs of success and progress. Being able to track progress, from one next best step to the next best step, is the motivator.

Lesson 3: Solution Focused thinking elevates conversations, practice, and change, taking it away from the identity problem. This is a chapter in a book with a specific focus on gender influencing work life as a Solution Focused practitioner, and I am saying sex and gender are not relevant. How is that for disruptive thinking?

Lesson 4: "trauma-informed" (Fallot & Harris, 2001) practices have their place in medical responses. They are not useful for whole-of-community responses to veteran and family support. Solution Focused practices affirm the veteran-centric policy goals that are meant to underpin all veteran support services. Veterans are the experts in what is working well for them, what their challenges are, and what they want their preferred future to be. Solutions that are co-designed are far more powerful and sustainable than a "one-size-fits-all" programme imposed by the "experts".

Which female practitioner inspires you and in which way?

There are three Solution Focused women I greatly admire and find inspirational. They have had a direct impact on the way I approach the work I do, and I am proud to call them colleagues and friends.

Lyn Worsley is a clinical psychologist and director of the Resilience Centre in Australia. It was Lyn who first introduced me to the world of Solution Focused practices. Every action in her practice is underpinned by the Solution Focused approach. Lyn walks the walk.

Emma Burns is a clinical psychologist working for the Police Department in New Zealand. The part of her work that inspires me is her Solution Focused practice bringing hope into some of the most challenging situations with her clients.

Annette Gray is a leadership coach, mentor, and facilitator in Australia. Her ability to use the Solution Focused approach to partner with clients using a genuinely client-led approach is inspirational in getting clients where they know they need to be.

What soft small notion would you encourage other women practitioners to embrace?

The small notion I encourage other women practitioners to embrace is "noticing and appreciating". Engaging this way instantly brings positivity, opens the mind to alternatives, and often creates motivation in very challenging situations. I want to encourage other practitioners to be more aware about the impact of language and the subtle way the choice of a word or the form of a question can change the course of a conversation and hence the exploration of new possibilities. Solution Focused practice is disruptive thinking. The best kind of disruptive thinking.

My best hopes for other female Solution Focused voices

My best hope for other female (and male) Solution Focused voices is that they recognise the opportunity Solution Focused practices can bring to all aspects of their professional life. It is a solid yet simple practice yielding powerful outcomes.

Co-constructive editors' reflections

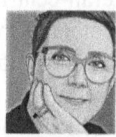 What I noticed in this chapter is Jacqui's clear belief that women are equal partners in society – it is a strong value for her. And I agree with her.

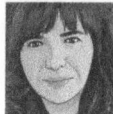 And in the veteran space she was told she was going to fail because she is not a veteran and because she is a woman; however, she turned it into an advantage because it allowed her to ask her clients and organisations difficult questions that would not normally be asked. This reminds me of Calyn Crow (2018, p. 155) saying that to discuss mental health and the military at the same time is nearly an "oxymoron". Jacqui is not too concerned about her gender; rather, she is more interested in authentic relationships and being authentic herself.

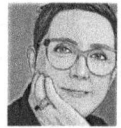 This authentic stance is related to the quote of "listening with the ear of your heart". And this might be a shift from empathy to compassion, as it has different nuances. I got this beautiful picture of a person with their heart standing out and it has small ears on it. This is a certain way of listening and I love that.

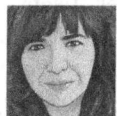 And I loved that she writes that wisdom and solutions come from the most unlikely sources. You really do not have to be the expert, as wisdom comes from such unlikely places. This once again makes me think of Crow (2018) saying how important it is to give control back to the veteran by accessing the ideas and tools they already have. And I loved that Jacqui said there was no room for playing the blame game, which reminds me of what Dawn Crosswhite and Johnny Kim (2018, p. 187) write about the Solution Focused approach and how it helps people "discover ways they have survived and strengths they have to move forward in their lives".

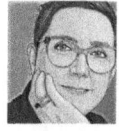 I loved it when she said the bulk of what we do is gathering people's stories of success. And I love that she said that the Solution Focused approach changes the energy in the conversation and that it is so hope transforming.

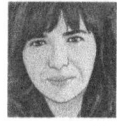 What really impressed me about this chapter is the idea that part of our job is to create disruptive thinking. It is about creating pattern interruptions in the problem narrative. And Jacqui challenges us by saying we need to disrupt thinking on a lot of levels – the client's narrative, the systems we work within, and even the way we help. She is saying we need to do things differently, which reminds me of Merritt Watson's (2018) book about her school, where she too wrote that we need to do differently on a lot of levels; we need to disrupt the old way of thinking.

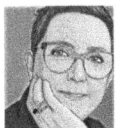

What I also noticed is that Jacqui clearly expressed that we move from "fixers to curious observers". When you are a curious observer you are stepping back and then you can be disruptive because your curiosity will lead to disruption. And I love that she says solutions are co-designed. I love this word, because it implies collaboration and uniqueness, as the design is different for each person. She is very passionate and determined about making changes in her society to disrupt the view of veterans in Australia.

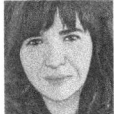

She talks about optimism, clarity, purpose, hope, motivation, encouragement, and expressing the truth. She likes the approach because it gives structure and boundaries, it keeps you on track, giving her direction or a "process" to follow (Froerer et al., 2018, p. 31). And I love that she notices and appreciates; this means she looks for what is working and going well and not re-traumatising her clients (Belous & Smith, 2018).

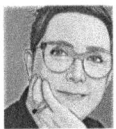

And I appreciated her mindfulness of the words and language she uses in her practice that changes the energy. One gets the impression her choice of words is a deliberate practice.

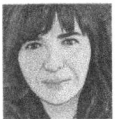

And I like that she shared that this way of working keeps her sane, which reminds me of vicarious resilience (Froerer et al., 2018), and I love that she said this approach gives the client control, especially when working with clients managing trauma (Reddy et al., 2018). Especially in the veteran space, where so much power has been taken away and the client feels so let down, Jacqui highlighted that the Solution Focused approach gives them back control and the power to choose how to manage and what to do next. That shows you are really coping with your life and, as Belous and Smith (2018, p, 225) state, increases "resilience and confidence".

Note

1   Benedict of Nursia, *Regula Sancti Benedicti* (AD 513), translated from the Latin: "et inclina aurem cordis tui".

Author reference

Fallot, R.D., & Harris, M. (2001). *Using trauma theory to design service systems*. Jossey-Bass.

Editor references

Belous, C., & Smith, C. (2018). Countering systemic retraumatization in sex trafficking. In A. Froerer, J. von Cziffra-Bergs, J. Kim & E. Connie (Eds.), *Solution Focused Brief Therapy and clients managing trauma*. Oxford University Press.

Crosswhite, D., & Kim, J. (2018). Child sexual abuse. In A. Froerer, J. von Cziffra-Bergs, J. Kim & E. Connie (Eds.), *Solution Focused Brief Therapy and clients managing trauma*. Oxford University Press.

Crow, C. (2018). Post traumatic stress disorder and the military. In A. Froerer, J. von Cziffra-Bergs, J. Kim & E. Connie (Eds.), *Solution Focused Brief Therapy and clients managing trauma*. Oxford University Press.

Froerer, A., von Cziffra-Bergs, J., Kim, J., & Connie, E. (2018). Vicarious resilience. In A. Froerer, J. von Cziffra-Bergs, J. Kim & E. Connie (Eds.), *Solution Focused Brief Therapy and clients managing trauma*. Oxford University Press.

Reddy, S., Bolton, K., Franklin, C., & Gonzalez Suitt, K. (2018). Substance abuse and recovery through SFBT. In A. Froerer, J. von Cziffra-Bergs, J. Kim & E. Connie (Eds.), *Solution Focused Brief Therapy and clients managing trauma*. Oxford University Press.

Watson, M. (2018). *Doing differently*. The Solution Focused Institute of South Africa.

Chapter 15

Infusing Solution Focused thinking within the New Zealand Police

Emma Burns (New Zealand)

Introduction

Solution Focused policing? Is there such a thing? I thought the Solution Focused approach was just for using in the therapy room! Perhaps that is what you believe too. It was certainly how I used to see the conversations I had with clients in my "pre-Solution Focused" life. However, learning this approach changed not only my work but my entire life as well. So my lifelong quest is to ask myself, "How can I bring the Solution Focused way of thinking and talking into other parts of my life?"

Reflect on how your gender influences your work–life and being a Solution Focused practitioner

Traditionally, the field of helping professionals has been predominantly female. Women are often regarded as having higher levels of patience, empathy, and compassion. From a very young age I have been drawn to those who are suffering or marginalised, advocated for them, and aspired to be a voice for the voiceless. The Solution Focused approach has given me a way of being able to advocate for people and ensure that their voices and hopes remain the loudest in the room.

I am a passionate advocate of the approach and strongly believe that it is a way of being, not just a method used at work. Solution Focused thinking has permeated my life, including my parenting, my relationships, and my own self-talk. When I first learned the approach, I was blessed to receive incredible support from experienced practitioners, both male and female colleagues. While this has not been universal (I have certainly experienced both overt and covert undermining and slander), I have never experienced being female as a barrier in any way.

Working for New Zealand Police, however, I discovered what it was like to be in a minority group. While the statistics have changed significantly since I joined in 2010, I began my role in two minority (and, arguably, less valued) groups: as a female and a non-sworn employee. As the only psychologist in the district, I was a sole practitioner, and had to create my own place within the organisation and earn the trust and respect of my colleagues. Discovering this approach one year later

DOI: 10.4324/9781003430254-16

gave me something that could benefit not only my clients but also my colleagues. Teaching police to utilise the approach in their work has been extremely rewarding, both to see the differences they can make with our customers and to witness the increased job satisfaction they enjoy as a result of experiencing different interactions and better relationships with the communities they serve.

What is your good reason for staying a Solution Focused practitioner?

As the Solution Focused tenet goes, if it ain't broke, don't fix it! Learning and practising the Solution Focused approach has transformed my work and changed my entire life. In my professional life, it has given me an optimistic outlook, a determination to find the good in a person (yes, even the worst offenders have wonderful traits and strengths), and the belief that they have the ability to create the life to which they aspire. This has also permeated my own life and transformed me from an extremely pessimistic and timid person into an optimistic, energetic, and more confident person who now has a genuine love for people. Additionally, I have seen the incredible difference that can be made when the approach is "mainstreamed" for use by members of the public. That is probably what I have become best known for doing in New Zealand.

Additionally, I love the positive ripple effect that this approach creates. Many people I have supported have gone on not only to successfully navigate future challenges but also to "pay it forward" to those around them. Two of my favourite examples are a grandmother who firmly believes two of her friends would no longer be alive had she not learned how to have helpful conversations, and a great young man I met in the police cells who was remanded in custody and proceeded to ask all his fellow "guests" the miracle question!

What would others notice you doing that would tell them that you work from a Solution Focused approach?

My colleagues hear me being curious about people and spending more time asking questions than making statements or drawing conclusions. When I first joined New Zealand Police, many of my colleagues wanted me to tell them why people did certain things and generally to "analyse" our customers (and sometimes their peers). It came as a disappointment to them that my usual response was, "I have no idea … I wonder what that person's reply to that question would be". I also do my best to avoid labels, preferring to stick to descriptions. This has no doubt been beneficial to my career, as it is much safer to talk about leaders who prefer frequent communication than to describe them as micromanagers.

They also hear me speaking about people's strengths and successes and reminding them that people do the best they can. This is very important in the world of policing, as my colleagues are dealing with people at their worst on their worst days, every single day they are at work. This can, understandably, result in them becoming cynical and ethically exhausted, and, at worst, beginning to dehumanise people. I believe that the mindset and narrative I bring to work have benefited my colleagues, providing them with a counter to what they experience and allowing them to hear the positive results we can achieve with those we help in the community.

I often suggest little "challenges" at work that secretly encourage colleagues to see our customers through a different lens. For example, I once ran a competition where each person had to discover the most interesting or impressive thing about someone they were working with (this could be a victim or an offender) and find out as much about that as possible. When we all shared what we had discovered, this was a powerful way of discovering a new way of seeing people. Positive gossip began replacing negative discourse about people, which led to an improved work culture.

For me, the way we see people is critical. One of my favourite quotes, which I include in my email signature, is "The way you see people is the way you treat them, and the way you treat them is what they become" (attributed to Johann Wolfgang von Goethe). I refer to this as maintaining a "benevolens", a word I made up that refers to a benevolent view of people that consciously and deliberately looks for the good, the valuable, and the admirable.

Finally, the most obvious clue for my colleagues would be my use of scaling and frequent utterance of the word "instead". I think that has become my favourite word, as it seamlessly shifts a conversation from being dominated by problems to one where hopes and possibilities can be discovered and grown.

However, my years of infecting New Zealand Police with the Solution Focused approach have not been without unintended consequences! On the rare occasions that I am having a not-so-good day, I can now expect various colleagues to ask me questions like, "If tomorrow is even a little bit better," "On a scale from 0 to 10 …" or "If you went to sleep tonight …". While this almost triggers a groan or an eye roll from me, it also delights me that they so naturally bring the Solution Focused approach into everyday conversations.

Share an exercise that might be useful to other female practitioners

I do not believe that Solution Focused is a gendered approach. That said, one of my favourite exercises to use in training is one I experienced when I attended a workshop facilitated by Annette Gray in 2022 for the Association for Coaching. Annette calls this exercise "You at Your Best" and people are asked to pair up with another person and given the following instructions:

- When you think of your best coaching conversations, what is it that works?
- What did you do that made it go so well?

While this exercise was focused on coaching conversations, it can easily be modified to include any kind of conversation or interaction, work-related or personal. I have used the activity to explore conversations that have gone better than expected with a wide range of audiences, from the general public to frontline professionals and senior leaders. In those examples, participants gave a brief description of the context, then focused specifically on what they had done that contributed to the success of the interaction. Upon returning to the larger group, each person spoke about what they had been impressed by in what they had heard. I find this to be a very simple yet powerful exercise that can be utilised both face to face or in an online setting.

I have also used this exercise several times as an opening activity with a variety of audiences as a gentle way of allowing people to experience the approach, and to give time at the beginning of a workshop to acknowledge and uplift the skills and experience that already exist in the room before commencing the training. For me, this is an activity that beautifully upholds the Solution Focused stance and is consistent with the Te Ao Māori principles mentioned later in this chapter.

Share how you adapt the approach and make it your own. Give us five characteristics that are a part of your Solution Focused DNA

When I first learned this approach, it was clear to me that this style of conversation held incredible power to make a difference for people, and that it was a beautifully respectful and encouraging way to be with people. Having been trained in clinical psychology, I often felt uncomfortable with many of the popular models that seemed to invite a hierarchical expert–client relationship. I found it a somewhat sterile communication style and it seemed to inherently dishonour the strengths and skills that clients brought with them. One of my favourite Te Ao Māori values is Kotahitanga, which relates to the importance of unity, true collaboration, and a shared vision. It is my belief that the Solution Focused approach upholds this and many other Te Ao Māori values, including Rangatiratanga, which refers to the importance of self-determination and the freedom to live one's life in a way that aligns with one's customs and values. For me this resonates with the statement attributed to Mahatma Gandhi, "What you do for me but without me, you do against me". Many Western models of therapy are perceived by people as being "done to" or imposed on them, whereas the Solution Focused approach represents a true partnership where the hopes and dreams of a person are supported, their strengths honoured, and their voice heard.

As mentioned earlier, I think I have adapted the approach to make it more accessible to nonclinical professionals and the general public. Because I see the Solution Focused approach as a way of thinking and talking about things, I do not believe this should remain solely the domain of clinicians. While there are clear differences between the groups, I absolutely believe that every person can benefit from learning how to have better conversations, including their own self-talk. To that end, I am probably best known in New Zealand as having "mainstreamed" the approach. My first experiences of "teaching" the approach was to a group of 130 members of the public who wanted to learn how to talk with those struggling with suicidal thoughts.

Many of the settings I work within neither want nor need to learn the approach in its entirety; people simply require a different way of doing things. I have developed several frameworks that I would describe as being "covert Solution Focused". These include the suicide prevention model S.A.F.E.™ (**S**ee, **A**sk, **F**ocus, **E**ncourage) and the interactional model H.E.L.P.™, which also includes a foundation of self-awareness and wellbeing for helping professionals (**H**ow Am I?, **E**ngagement, **L**istening with Curiosity, **P**artnering for Solutions). One of the early workshops was with a large group of men on Men's Health Week at a local pub. To fit the theme and venue, we talked about how beer can save a life (**B**e Aware, **E**nquire, **E**ncourage, **R**efocus)! My love of acronyms makes me wonder if I am institutionalised after having worked for New Zealand Police for nearly 13 years.

Which female practitioner inspires you and in which way?

I hold many of my colleagues in extremely high regard for various reasons. However, if I had to choose just one woman, it would have to be Eve Lipchik. I first became aware of Eve when I stumbled across her 2014 article, "The development of my personal Solution-Focused working model: From 1978 and continuing". Reading this was like a breath of fresh air, as someone was finally talking about emotions, empathy, and relationships. I often feel that discussions about the Solution Focused approach become heavily theoretical and focus exclusively on technique, and consequently the relationship with the client, and indeed the client themselves, is lost. I went on to read her book *Beyond technique in Solution-Focused therapy: Working with emotions and the therapeutic relationship*, which, needless to say, only cemented my admiration and respect for Eve. Since that time, I have been inspired by several of her other writings and was incredibly honoured to be one of the people who spoke with her in a webinar hosted by Family Based Solutions in February 2021.

I am aware that many in our Solution Focused community do not believe that empathy or relationships are important factors. While I respect their opinions, I could not agree less. In my experience working with marginalised groups and those who are rejected by society at large, empathy and building relationships (known as Whakawhanaungatanga in Te Reo Māori) are vital ingredients. This was abundantly clear to me when I developed my project working with those in police custody. My experience was that empathy was the magical ingredient that broke down barriers, established trust, and opened up deep and sacred conversations. This cemented my belief that empathy and a trusting relationship are critical ingredients for any helping conversation. For me empathy, emotions, and relationships are paramount, while techniques are very much secondary.

What soft small notion would you encourage other women practitioners to embrace?

Solution Focused practice is often described as a way of listening, and there are many well-known quotes about listening being more important than speaking.

While, of course, questions are important in encouraging people to think in a different way, we cannot ask good questions if we are not listening well. However, we often forget that listening includes listening to ourselves; not only listening to ourselves speak out loud but also listening to the small voice within us. Some may call that voice a gut feeling, some may call it intuition or inner wisdom, but our inner voice is a gift as valuable as – albeit often less valued than – our audible voice.

Never become so caught up in technique, specific questions, or desired outcomes that you lose connection with your inner voice or intuition. Learn to slow down and be in the moment with people. To that end, I have included references to some of my favourite writings by Eve Lipchik. Whenever you find yourself feeling clever or excessively focusing on theory or technique, go and make a cup of coffee, sit down, and read some of these.

My best hopes for other female Solution Focused voices

Never let anyone intimidate you or make you think you aren't clever enough, educated enough, old enough, experienced enough, liberal enough, or any of the other "enoughs". If you love the approach and are passionate about using it to make the world a better place for those around you, don't listen to anyone who tries to put you down or make things difficult for you.

Unfortunately, you may come across people in the Solution Focused world who will take any opportunity to discredit you or criticise what you do. As Shakespeare said, "To thine own self be true". Never stop learning, but remember that your clients are your best teachers. New versions of the approach will come and go, but the tenets that underpin the approach will remain. Hold fast to those, maintain your love for people and for your work, and you will succeed.

And if anyone ever needs encouragement, I would love to support you!

Co-constructive editors' reflection

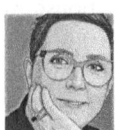

What was so amazing reading this chapter was that Emma is a voice for the voiceless. This is really beautiful and frames the whole chapter. She talked about how the Solution Focused approach is a way of being and it made me think that we wrote about **being** Solution Focused in the first chapter but never mentioned it to the contributors, yet it has been a common thread to talk about **being** Solution Focused. I think when we find the Solution Focused approach to be a perfect match it is because it resonates with some of our embedded values as a person.

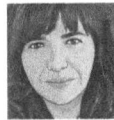

Yes, and I loved how Emma is a voice for her client's hopes and that she is blessed to be Solution Focused, almost as though it is a gift to **be** Solution Focused. Emma also mentioned that, working in the police, she now knows what it is like to be a minority and she can relate to what it is like to be marginalised. And this strengthens her resolve to be a voice of hope for the voiceless. What really stood out for me is how Emma mentioned that the Solution Focused Approach can be mainstreamed and is not just a therapeutic approach. She says it has a positive ripple effect and that we can use this approach everywhere with everyone. Just like Harriet Conniff saying it is like a "Solution Focused injection" (2021, p. 111).

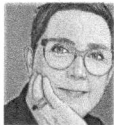 Yes, and I agree with her. I think she is right; we need to think about how we can take the approach into the larger community.

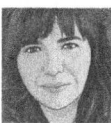 Emma reminds us of a key factor in the Solution Focused approach, which is to ask questions rather than being the expert. She is not an expert about anything and would rather be curious and ask a question. This made me think of Barnai and Soregi (2021, p.130) saying the right question "opens a gateway to powerful new thinking". Emma is also constantly aware of the fact that people do the best they can in life; as Harriet Conniff (2021, p. 109) says, not seeing people as "failing" but just trying to get through their life and having "good reasons for how they behave" (Barnai & Soregi, 2021, p. 133).

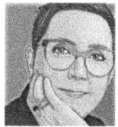 Emma is constantly empathic, even with her colleagues, and understands that they deal with people on the worst day of their lives, and she stays empathic and hopeful. I love that she says she works with hope, joy, and optimism (Burns, 2021).

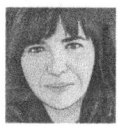 And that talking and being hopeful is nearly a counter-experience, a counterbalance to all the harsh negativities. She even encourages positive gossip in a determined, persistent way – so much so that her colleagues even start Solution talking back to her. It reminds me of Merritt Watson saying, "We want an institution filled with joy and happiness" (Birkett & Watson, 2021, p. 88) where positivity can spread.

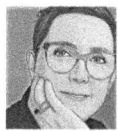 Yes, it was really fun, almost like payback time. And makes me think that this way of being in the world rubs off positively.

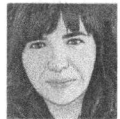 I loved the way Emma made up her own word "benevolens" because it underlines how she values looking at people at their best. It reminded me of how I often talk about a "Soulution" Focused lens (von Cziffra-Bergs, 2018) and how we need to focus on really seeing people and not the crisis or the offence.

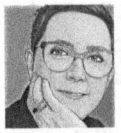 This also reminded me of how we collect metaphors in the Solution Focused approach and how we use language very playfully. And I loved her simple, useful, and transferable exercise. We can generalise it for any situation.

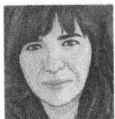 What stands out for me is the simplicity and the power of generalising that Emma brings to the approach, nothing fancy or complicated; just simplistic in the power of making a difference. She is very aware of seeing her clients as her partners. She does not call her clients co-experts but rather partners, which is personal and intimate – it has a togetherness connection. And that the conversation is a sacred emotional conversation, which is what partners do.

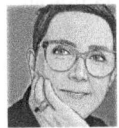 And this is her natural authentic way of being with people, coming from her heart. And it reminds me of doing Solution Focused with a soft touch. Emma reminds us that our inner voice, intuition, authentic self, or gut should be the leading star, rather than techniques. And I think this is nice to think about – slow down and listen to our inner voice, really beautiful!

Author references

Lipchik, E. (1993). The integration of emotion in Solution-Focused therapy. *Journal of Marital and Family Therapy*, *19*(3), 233–242.

Lipchik, E. (2011). *Beyond technique in Solution-Focused therapy: Working with emotions and the therapeutic relationship*. The Guilford Press.

Lipchik, E. (2014). The development of my personal Solution-Focused working model: From 1978 and continuing. *International Journal of Solution-Focused Practices*, *2*(2), 63–73.

Editor references

Barnai, A., & Soregi, V. (2021). Facing new challenges using the Solution Focused approach: Creating a supportive learning process for Roma adolescents in a volunteering project in Hungary. In D. Yusuf (Ed.), *The Solution Focused approach with children and young people*. Routledge.

Birkett, N., & Watson, M. (2021). Dream … believe … achieve: A school in South Africa that has developed a philosophy based on Solution Focused principles. In D. Yusuf (Ed.), *The Solution Focused approach with children and young people*. Routledge.

Burns, E. (2021). Using the Solution Focused approach within the New Zealand Police to create happy endings for young people and their families. In D. Yusuf (Ed.), *The Solution Focused approach with children and young people*. Routledge.

Conniff, H. (2021). Solution Focused "injections": Solution Focused working in acute paediatric settings. In D. Yusuf (Ed.), *The Solution Focused approach with children and young people*. Routledge.

von Cziffra-Bergs, J. (2018). SFBT and violent crime. In A. Froerer, J. von Cziffra-Bergs, J. Kim & E. Connie (Eds.), *Solution Focused Brief Therapy and clients managing trauma*. Oxford University Press.

Chapter 16

Breaking bars and building dreams

A female psychologist's perspectives on working in a male prison

Zibeth Hansen (South Africa)

Introduction

I am a clinical psychologist working in a correctional setting (prison) in South Africa. The facility at which I work is about 100 km north of Cape Town and has three centres, with a total of around 1,500 offenders. Although I primarily render services to about 800 male offenders in the maximum-security centre, I also work at the juvenile and medium-security centres from time to time. The offenders I encounter daily have mostly been convicted of serious violent and sexual offences and are serving lengthy prison sentences. About a quarter of these offenders are serving life or even multiple life sentences. I am in awe of how talented, creative, and resourceful these guys are – they can build the most detailed and carefully crafted model ships from matches. When the choir performs at internal events, you always want to hear just one more song. These examples do not even begin to describe the talents and ingenuity of these men.

Reflect on how your gender influences your work–life and being a Solution Focused practitioner

It is a harsh man's world in a male correctional facility or prison. As a woman working in a male maximum-security correctional facility, not only are all my clients male but so are most of the officials with whom I work. I had to learn how to navigate the unique environmental and interpersonal dynamics in this male-dominated, para-militaristic security setting. This environment is often perceived as harsh, hostile, difficult, and intimidating. Many of my supervisors and lecturers tried to persuade me to pick an alternative field of focus because "prison is not a place for a woman". I, however, enjoy working with offenders and believe it is the perfect environment for me. Although I do not see myself as someone who draws particular attention to my womanhood through hair, nails, or make-up, for example, I do believe that I bring something different, something more feminine, to the situation, which inevitably changes the interactional dynamics of this male-dominated environment.

DOI: 10.4324/9781003430254-17

When people hear that I work in a prison they are either appalled or intrigued, but always curious about what I do and about the offenders with whom I work. I am often asked whether I am scared of working with these (dangerous) offenders, many of whom are incarcerated for violent and sexual offences against women and children. People are also curious about how I can interact with these men, knowing what they have done, and not be repulsed. For me the answer to these questions is simple: No, I am not afraid of being with them because I see them as humans who are much more than the offence they have committed. They each have a voice that needs to be heard and a story that needs to be listened to and understood. I do believe that, as a woman, I have a unique opportunity not only to intervene in terms of criminogenic needs and offence-supporting attitudes but also, through the therapeutic relationship, to foster and model what appropriate relationships with boundaries and interactions with women should look like.

When I started my journey as a psychologist, I knew that I wanted to work in the forensic setting, but I did not see myself as a therapist, since none of the therapeutic approaches really resonated with me. I always thought I would focus more on court assessments and reports. This was until I was appropriately introduced to Solution Focused therapy at a workshop by Dr Jacqui von Cziffra-Bergs. The approach reso-nated with me not only as a psychologist but also through who I am as a person and my inherent view of people and the world; and by default my view of offenders and correcting offending behaviour. Since then, I have been able to define and hone my skills as a therapist, and now I really enjoy the therapeutic interactions and am privileged to see the progress some of these offenders make during therapy and beyond the termination of the therapeutic process.

What is your good reason for staying a Solution Focused practitioner?

The primary aim of most prison facilities is rehabilitation through identifying and intervening in criminogenic needs (factors that contribute to offending behaviour) in order to address the offending behaviour and reduce the risk of recidivism and re-offending. Most programmes and interventions focus on the problems, limita-tions, mistakes, and faults of individual offenders. In essence, these programmes establish what went wrong in the past, what is wrong at present, and what might go wrong in the future that made this offender commit the offence or may contribute to him committing a similar offence. In addition, considering the socio-economic climate of South Africa, many of these offenders come from impoverished back-grounds where substance abuse, family violence, public violence, gangsterism, and crime are the order of the day.

Once you start focusing on these problems and challenges, it is easy to become overwhelmed and experience feelings of hopelessness and powerlessness. The environment and interaction quickly become problem saturated. This often results in burnout not only among psychologists, social workers, and other professionals in the system but also among custodial officials tasked with the day-to-day care of offenders.

In my experience, working from a Solution Focused perspective protects me from burnout because, while I still have to identify the criminogenic needs, I also identify each offender's strengths and use this in therapy. It also protects me against vicarious traumatisation, as Solution Focused therapy allows me to identify areas of intervention without requiring me to delve into the details of the (sometimes horrific) crimes or the offender's own past trauma. This approach allows therapy to shift from a past and problem focus to a future and Solution Focus, which automatically creates a sense of hopefulness among the offenders. While incarcerated offenders often feel that they have limited agency, working from a Solution Focused perspective gives them a sense of control over their future, even for those who serve long sentences. In my experience, being involved in a Solution Focused process allows offenders to change their concept of the "future". This is especially helpful for offenders who are serving long determinate sentences, or even life sentences, where they may be incarcerated for the bigger part of what is left of their natural lives. Some of these definition shifts include, for example, that their "future" is making sure that their children do not engage in criminal behaviour or become involved with gangs, causing them to end up in prison themselves. Envisioning a better future for their loved ones is often the motivation these offenders use to make changes to their own lives.

What would others notice you doing that would tell them that you work from a Solution Focused approach?

The Solution Focused approach is more than just a way of conducting therapy; it is a way of being, living, and interacting. I believe that others will notice this way of being in my general approach to the correctional system and particularly offenders, through my actions and the language I choose to use. I choose to see the person and not the prisoner. I always treat offenders with the same respect and dignity as I would any other person, regardless of the reason for their incarceration or the seriousness of their offence. I truly believe that I cannot expect someone to be better if I do not treat them better. I cannot help someone to be their best possible self if I judge and treat them based on their worse decisions and actions. I also avoid negative labelling and derogatory language as far as possible when speaking to or about offenders. In addition, I never call offenders by their gang or street names, despite them often being referred to by those names in the centre, but choose to call them by their given names in an attempt to help them establish a future identity that is tangibly different from the identity they associate with their offending behaviour.

Maybe what others will notice is best summarised in this excerpt from a poem by one of the offenders I saw in therapy:

> *I am grateful for her strength and integrity to come to this place*
> *Some say it is dark, others say it is hell*

But for her it is a river of flowing waters – something like a well
She always manages a smile no matter how bad the day
This is my psychologist! If I must say
Thank you for kindness
Thank you for honesty
For never judging, and always believing in me
Without her coming around – I don't know where I would be!

By no means do I think that I am doing anything extraordinary, but what I have learned is that treating offenders with dignity and giving them back their humanity goes a long way in making a big difference. Working from a Solution Focused perspective affords me the incomparable opportunity to create a therapeutic space, and interact with offenders in a way that is in sharp contrast to the rest of the prison environment they experience.

Share an exercise that might be useful to other women practitioners

The skill of listening with a Solution Focused ear

People, especially offenders, are very good at complaining, detailing their problems, and highlighting everything that is wrong. In essence, they are very good at being problem rather than solution focused. As such, one of the most valuable Solution Focused skills I have learned (and that I am still refining) is to listen with a different, Solution Focused ear. An ear that can hear the hidden strengths, values, goals, and future hopes that are at the core of the complaint or problem the offender brings into the therapeutic space. Once you are able to hear those positive qualities and reflect them back to the offender using positive and/or presuppositional Solution Focused language, it changes the dynamic of any therapeutic interaction. Offenders automatically become less resistant and combative. They feel valued and understood, which ensures their buy-in into the collaborative therapeutic process.

The excerpt below is based on a conversation I had with an offender who had been referred for a suicide risk evaluation and therapy. He was frustrated and angry when he came into the session. I encourage you to read through it and see how good you are at listening with your Solution Focused ear.

I am not happy with how things are going at the prison. They refuse to assist me with the things that I am complaining about. I completed a Home-Based Carer Course in August, but they spelled my name wrong on the certificate. They said that they'll correct it, [but] it is now March and they still haven't given me my new certificate. This upsets me because I had a 100% attendance and wanted to learn new skills. I told the instructor that I will rather be dead than live under these rules and conditions. I did not say that I was going to kill myself, they misunderstood me. Now I am on suicide watch, and I don't want to be on it. I am not crazy. I have nothing to do during the day. I just sit in my cell. I have asked for work, but they don't want to give me a job in the prison. I used to do needle-work. I fixed clothes and pillows and embroidered patterns on them. Because they think I want to kill myself, they have now taken away my needles and I am not allowed to do it anymore. I also want to transfer to a prison closer to home and my mother and daughter. This prison is too far away, and they cannot visit me. I want to go back to Gauteng so that I can see them. I have not gotten any feedback on any of the transfer requests that I have made. All I ever hear from these people are empty promises.

When you listen with a problem-focused ear, you might feel overwhelmed, power-less, and hopeless about this offender's situation. But how many strengths were you able to identify while listening with your Solution Focused ear? What can you reflect back to him? Maybe that he is hardworking? Maybe that his relationship with his family is important to him? Maybe that he is motivated to develop him-self? What else? Start training your Solution Focused ear by doing this exercise in everyday conversations. When people complain, try to listen for the strengths and values that they are inadvertently sharing with you.

Share how you adapt the approach and make it your own. Give us five characteristics that are a part of your Solution Focused DNA

Working as a psychologist in the correctional system, I have three main professional responsibilities, the first of which are interventions aimed at improving the general and overall mental health of offenders. This aspect includes the usual responsibil-ities associated with working as a psychologist, such as identifying and treating those presenting with emotional distress, suicidality, or symptoms associated with mental health conditions related to mood, anxiety, trauma, etc. In addition, I render rehabilitative psycho-therapeutic services where intervention is aimed at the crim-inogenic needs of offenders, as explained in the preceding sections. Lastly, I con-duct risk assessments and provide reports to the parole board commenting on the offender's re-offending risk level once they qualify for parole consideration. The last two areas are unique to the correctional environment, so I will elaborate on how I have adapted and utilised the Solution Focused approach in these two areas.

I want to start this off with a disclaimer – I am not a Solution Focused purist, but rather an eclectic therapist who works from a Solution Focused frame of reference. That being said, I feel that the Solution Focused approach is easily integrated with rehabilitative work because of its future-focused perspective. No offender wants to return to prison, so I usually ask them what they think needs to change in their lives to enable them to live a life that does not cycle back to offending behaviour and incarceration. This helps them to collaboratively identify rehabilitative goals and gives us a point of departure for therapy. In addition, there are also evidence-based offender treatment models, such as the Good Lives Model (GLM), supported by a wealth of empirical evidence that can easily be integrated with Solution Focused therapy. The GLM still identifies criminogenic needs but approaches these from a positive psychology rather than a psychopathology perspective.

Initially, it was a bit more difficult for me to incorporate my Solution Focused approach into the risk assessment part of my work because risk assessments, by default, are designed to identify problem areas that may increase an offender's risk for future re-offending. I, however, choose to assess not only risk areas but also protective factors (strengths) that may reduce an offender's risk for future re-offending. This technique allows me to present a balanced view of the offender that gives hope and highlights strengths that may act as a buffer against recidivism, while also acknowledging the risk areas that still need to be addressed. I further-more choose to give feedback on these assessments to the offenders in a way that commends them on the progress towards rehabilitation that they have made thus far. I also give them positive feedback about their strengths and the areas on which they can focus to further reduce their risk of re-offending.

Which female practitioner inspires you and in which way?

I have a lot of respect for and draw a lot of inspiration from the work of Marjan Gryson and Veerle De Waele, associated with VZW Touché. They have done some amazing Solution Focused work with incarcerated offenders in Belgium in terms of reducing aggressive and violent behaviour. Their aim is not to eradicate the aggression, but rather to teach offenders how to channel it positively into a motiv-ating, creative, and constructive, rather than a destructive, force. They refer to this as positive aggression.

Anger management programmes often teach offenders to avoid situations or interactions that might lead to feelings of anger and aggressive behaviour. Anger is unintentionally labelled as an emotion to avoid at all costs. The work of these two phenomenal women teaches offenders that anger is a normal emotion that can even be seen as a strength when it is embraced and channelled correctly. I think it is extremely important to teach offenders to recognise, embrace, and constructively use their emotions, especially those that are perceived as negative. This is probably one of the most important skills with which to address reactive violence.

What soft small notion would you encourage other women practitioners to embrace?

We all have a natural intuitive sense that picks up subtle cues from our environ-ment and from those with whom we interact directly or indirectly. Although most therapists, regardless of gender, are aware of this, I do believe that as women we are naturally intuitive. We often have that "gut feeling" we can't quite explain or provide concrete reasons for – we just have this sense. Whether it signals danger, or discomfort, or a question that pops up in your mind during therapy that seems to be only vaguely related to the discussion at hand, or anything else. Sometimes we ignore that "gut feeling" because, in a world that values tangible facts, we are often made to feel that intuition is second rate. People tend to become conditioned to ignore their gut feelings. If there is one small notion that I would encourage women to embrace not just in therapy but also in their life in general, it would be to embrace and trust that gut feeling.

My best hopes for other female Solution Focused voices

My wens is eenvoudig, ek wil sien dat vroulike stemme in die Solution Focused gemeenskap meer prominent word. Vroue doen ongelooflike werk en maak 'n groot verskil in verskeie gemeenskappe en instellings, maar meestal word die werk in stilte gedoen. Ek hoop dat hierdie boek as 'n platform sal dien wat ander vroue sal aanmoedig om hulle stories en ervarings te deel en by ons stories te las. Ek hoop dat daar 'n tyd sal kom waar elke vrou sal besef dat hul storie en hul ervaring die moeite werd is om gedeel en gehoor te word. Ongeag hoe sag hulle dink hul stem is. Ek sien uit daarna dat vroue stemme van regoor die wêreld saamspan in 'n ondersteunende gemeenskap waar eendersdenkende vroue kan deel met mekaar, kan leer van mekaar, en mekaar kan ondersteun.

My best hope is simple – I would love to hear female voices speak up in the Solution Focused community. Women are doing incredible work in a variety of settings and making huge differences in communities and settings, but this is often done in silence. I hope that this book serves as a platform that sparks other phenomenal women to add their voices and their stories to ours. My hope is that every woman realises that their voice and their story deserve to be heard, no matter how small they think their voice might be. I would love to see female voices joined together in a supportive community where like-minded women can share, learn, and feel supported.

Author's reflection

When I was initially asked to contribute to this project, I was excited but also felt that my voice is such a small one in a sea of amazing voices from around the world, and I was not sure if it was truly a voice in which others would be interested. Reflecting on the process of writing this contribution, I realised that so many women feel that their voices and contributions are small and limited, and therefore they never make themselves heard. I am honoured to have shared my voice with the world and hope that it can inspire others to follow suit. The process of writing this chapter reminded me once again of how much I enjoy the work that I do, and how lucky I am to live my passion every day. It has also reignited a best hope and personal aspiration that had been pushed aside when the world's focus shifted towards COVID, namely to develop a Solution Focused therapeutic group intervention programme aimed at addressing the needs of offenders that is specific to the South African context, rather than programmes that have been adapted from Eurocentric research and treatments.

Co-constructive editors' reflection

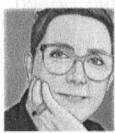 This chapter was such a pleasure. She works in this special setting, and clearly states, "I am not afraid of being with them because I see them as humans who are much more than the offence they have committed". They each have a voice that needs to be heard and a story that needs to be listened to and understood.

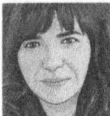 I underlined exactly that line as well. I loved when she said, "I'm able to foster and model appropriate relationships, boundaries, and interactions with women and what they should look like," but she's modelling way more. There's a lot of modelling on so many levels. She models how to view people, how to connect with people, to other colleagues how to treat people, and to her clients how to treat women.

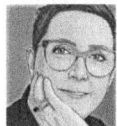 You're right, this view of hers can be seen on so many levels. It's clear she has ideas about how this can be done and what it should look like. She is on a kind of mission of showing it to people. She is so deliberate in her choice of working from this stance and saying *this is the best way for me to not get burnt out*. It is evident not only on a therapeutic level in her relationship with offenders but also with colleagues and, yes, in her life as a whole.

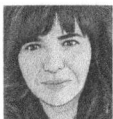 Zibeth is very aware that, in the offender context, the focus is on what went wrong and on how to prevent things from going wrong again, which is not hopeful. She sees it as her job to create a balance between problem talk. This reminds me of what Carla Smith and Christopher Belous (2018, p. 218) write – saying that she always asks questions, or adds phrases and statements that "incite resilience for the client".

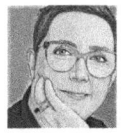 And Zibeth has this idea about moving away from the past and the problem to the future, and maybe there is no solution for the future, but how do we want life to be or how could it look like in the best possible way under those conditions? And I really love how the Solution Focused approach allows offenders to change their concept of the future. There is still a future, no matter how immediately hopeless it may look.

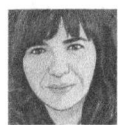 What I love is shifting the future by making sure that their children don't engage in criminal activity. It nearly becomes like those relationship questions – a systemic change that will impact not only the client's life but also the betterment of their children. Envisioning a better future for their loved ones is often the motivation these offenders need to change their own lives. She also says, "I choose to see the person and not the prisoner", which reminds me of Dawn Crosswhite (2018, p. 94), who writes that she treats all people "with worth and potential". Zibeth talks to her clients by using their given names. And then one of her clients responded with the most beautiful poem.

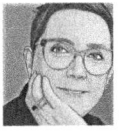

That's right. She sees them as people, not as gang members, but individuals, which is why she uses their names. I think it is beautiful, and it's a small difference that makes a difference.

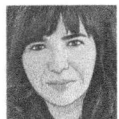

And I have learned that treating offenders with dignity, giving them back their humanity goes a long way. And I think the poem is a reflection of a client who has experienced her doing that.

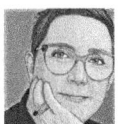

It is a statement of "This is my psychologist", a really strong statement, said with a kind of pride.

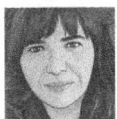

Yes, and then she says it gives her an incredible opportunity to create a space and to interact in sharp contrast to the rest of prison life. She really makes a contrasting experience for them. It's like the therapeutic space is an exception to the rule of everyday life. It's not only an exception; it's a magic transforming opportunity place.

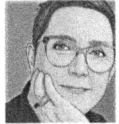

And what she writes about creating a balanced view of the offender reminds me about the Signs of Safety, because I think that is exactly what she is doing. It's a balanced assessment and Zibeth also balances her view about the offender, between strengths, possibilities, skills, and competences and not only concerns about recidivism.

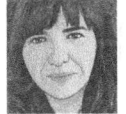

And what I also loved is where she said, this balanced view of giving a bit of hope and then highlighting strengths, acts as a buffer to the possibility of falling back. Then something she wrote that made me very interested and tickled my interest, because I have never heard of positive aggression.

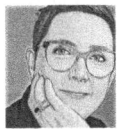

Marjan Gryson and Veerle De Waele from Belgium have presented at an EBTA conference in Bruges on their work within prisons; it's very impressive.

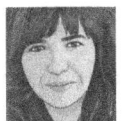

She has realised that the aim is not to eradicate aggression, but to shift it into a constructive force rather than a destructive one. I love that because it's about channelling it correctly. It's about embracing their emotions.

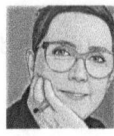 And she mentioned this gut feeling and I think there are no words to describe what it is. We all know this in-between space in therapy. I think to embrace and trust that, whether it's intuition or a gut feeling, is so important and so beautiful. "If there's one small notion that I would encourage women to embrace, it is to embrace and trust that gut feeling" – that's actually a really beautiful quote.

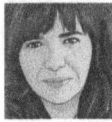 And in a world that often values tangible facts, we are often made to believe that intuition is second-rate. This correlates with what Calyn Crow (2018, p. 176) writes, saying "we have to start trusting the guide within us".

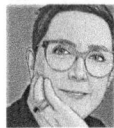 I also love her Best Hopes, and her personal reflections were beautiful. The process that she's describing in her reflection, moving from *I was just considering doing what every woman would do, not writing this chapter because I don't have a voice that is strong enough or significant enough or …* But, no way! I'm writing this chapter because my voice is just as important as anybody else's. It was lovely to read her thought process and her reflections and see how writing this chapter has empowered her.

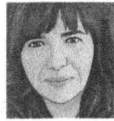 Many women feel their voices and contributions are small, or limited, and therefore they never make themselves heard. That's how she felt and the mere act of writing the chapter is showing us her journey and her courage and her taking it on.

Author references

Barnao, M., Ward, T., & Robertson, P. (2016). The Good Lives Model: A new paradigm for forensic mental health. *Psychiatry, Psychology and Law*, *23*(2), 288–301. http://dx.doi.org/10.1080/13218719.2015.1054923

Clause, H., Beyens, K., De Meyer, R., Gryson, M, & Naessens, L. (2017). *The houses: Towards a sustainable penitentiary approach.* Vwz De Huizen.

Dealey, J. (2018). Moving beyond the risk paradigm: Using the Good Lives Model with offenders in denial of sexual offending. *European Journal of Probation*, *10*(1), 28–42. https://doi.org/10.1177/2066220318755530

Fortune, C. (2018). The Good Lives Model: A strength-based approach for youth offenders. *Aggression and Violent Behaviour*, *38*(Jan–Feb), 21–30. https://doi.org/10.1016/j.avb.2017.11.003

Gryson, M., & De Waele, V. (2017). *Positief agressief – Hoe woede benutten?* VZW Touche Institute. www.vzwtouche.be/nl

Hansen, Z., & Joubert, J. (2018). Solution building in South African correctional centres. In J. von Cziffra-Bergs (Ed.), *Creative solution building: Solution Focused Brief Therapy across Southern Africa* (pp. 153–173). Solution Focused Institute of South Africa.

Yates, P.M., & Prescott, D.S. (2011). *Building a better life: A Good Lives and Self-Regulation workbook.* The Safer Society Press.

Yates, P.M., Prescott, D., & Ward, T. (2010). *Applying the Good Lives and Self-Regulation models to sex offender treatment: A practical guide for clinicians.* The Safer Society Press.

Editor references

Belous, C., & Smith, C. (2018). Countering systemic retraumatization in sex trafficking. In A. Froerer, J. von Cziffra-Bergs, J. Kim & E. Connie (Eds.), *Solution Focused Brief Therapy and clients managing trauma*. Oxford University Press.

Crosswhite, D., and Kim, J. (2018). Interpersonal violence. In A. Froerer, J. Von Cziffra-Bergs, J. Kim & E. Connie (Eds.), *Solution Focused Brief Therapy and clients managing trauma*. Oxford University Press.

Crow, C. (2018). Post traumatic stress disorder and the military. In A. Froerer, J. von Cziffra-Bergs, J. Kim & E. Connie (Eds.), *Solution Focused Brief Therapy and clients managing trauma*. Oxford University Press.

Chapter 17

Empowering women survivors of violence at domestic violence shelters using an SFBT lens

Experiences of a Muslim woman practitioner

Zubeda Dangor (South Africa)

Introduction

I am a clinical psychologist who is privileged to work primarily in spaces with women and girls. After completing my PhD, my thesis was published in a book called *Life after abuse: An exploration of women's strategies for overcoming abuse*. I am passionate about helping women transform their lives for the better. I know that alone I cannot change the world, which is in desperate need of change, but I can, as Mother Teresa once said, "cast a stone across the waters to create many ripples" (Book, 2023). I therefore started the Nisaa Institute of Women's Development, a non-governmental organisation that offers shelter and places of safety for women.

Reflect on how your gender influences your work–life and being a Solution Focused practitioner

Growing up as a young Muslim woman in apartheid-era South Africa, I felt under-valued and disrespected. It was not until I was pursuing a master's degree in psychology that I realised how silent I had become and that I had never spoken up compared to my classmates. A defining moment for me was when one of my female lecturers encouraged me to speak up. She kept saying that she knew I had potential and that she valued my insights, and she kept challenging me to use my voice and share my ideas. This experience changed my life, and through my personal experience I realised that there had to be many other women who are disempowered and remain silent.

After I received my master's degree, I spent six months in the United States, studying violence against women. When I came back, I started a research project on women in the south of Johannesburg who experience domestic violence. Here I worked with a male colleague who demanded that he be the first author of our article, who kept rejecting my knowledge and elevating his name. When a German organisation came to South Africa and funded the research, one of the funders, a German woman, told me to stand up for myself – she said that his behaviour was unacceptable and she would only deal with me. I was shocked at the time that a

DOI: 10.4324/9781003430254-18

woman would stand up for another woman. It completely empowered me, and I found my voice. I felt heard and valued on multiple levels and decided not to give up my opinion, knowledge, passion, and justice for people. I always ask myself, "What are you going to do about it, how do you want things to be different?" and I decided to accept the challenge and not allow anyone to oppress me ever again. My deep personal experiences have motivated me to make a difference in other women's lives.

As a woman, I feel privileged to work especially in areas with women and girls, as I believe that women are "the largest untapped reservoir of talent in the world" (Hillary Clinton, as quoted in Ha, 2017), which they often fail to recognise because society views women as oppressed. The high level of gender-based violence (Gouws, 2022) in South Africa and the lack of adequate services for women inspire me to work with women to empower them to overcome their oppression and see themselves as empowered beings with dignity and self-respect.

This is also why I started a women's shelter organisation. At the women's shelter, we see that women live in silence, with shame and guilt, thinking that violence only happens to them. I believe that if we break the silence and start building friendships and support, they can regain their lives. I know that it is my purpose – to serve as a catalyst for women. I offer them an opportunity, a safe space, huge respect, and multicultural understanding, and invite them to start dreaming about a new future. I believe that they are people with their own goals and that their goals are not my goals or the shelter's goals but their own personal goals for a different life.

What is your good reason for staying a Solution Focused practitioner?

The Solution Focused approach aligns with my belief system as a Muslim woman and my own approach to psychotherapy. Islam has recognised mental health issues since the eighth century. It acknowledges mental wellbeing as an integral part of overall health. Islam's emphasis on compassion, empathy, and caring for oneself and others sets the foundation for addressing mental health and acknowledging that mental distress can affect a person's ability to fulfil religious and societal duties (M. Mangera, personal communication, August 2023). I come from an Islamic belief system, and we learn from a famous narration of Prophet Mohamed (PBUH) "who so-ever knows himself knows his Lord" (Isgandarova, 2017, p. 253). The concept of "Nafs" (the self or psyche) is intricately interwoven into Islamic teaching, highlighting the importance of nurturing a balanced and peaceful state of mind. The Prophet's (PBUH) compassion for those experiencing emotional distress, his encouragement to seek advice, and his recognition of human vulnerability underscore Islam's understanding of the complexities of mental health, which is also part of Solution Focused Brief Therapy (M. Mangera, personal communication, August 2023).

The Solution Focused approach allows me to help my clients know themselves and not only their past violence. The Prophet Mohamed's (PBUH) teachings on removing harm from others and his affirmation that faith is rooted in the heart's tranquillity highlight the significance of addressing emotional pain. Islam's holistic approach to wellbeing encompasses emotional, physical, and spiritual health. Seeking counselling aligns with the latter approach, fostering healing, resilience, and a stronger connection with Allah (God).

The Solution Focused approach allows me to harness positivity in approaching my clients and not pathologise or negatively label them. Labelling does not allow a person to see internal struggles as an opportunity for growth.

An important reason for staying Solution Focused is that this approach invites people into the future, and when one has been abused and belittled one forgets about the possibility of a different future. What I often experience during my work is that women may be stuck in a problem-focused, negative narrative. This makes them feel more vulnerable and helpless and does not allow them to feel in control of themselves or able to find the solutions they seek. However, "the future is entirely what each one of us does every day", to quote Gloria Steinem (Equality Now, 2020). This aligns not only with my Solution Focused lens but also with my Islamic view that we are creators of our own reality. We can make choices that are different to the ones we previously made. Solution Focused practice provides a vehicle for me to achieve my goals and a methodology that guides my engagement and practice, without interfering with my spiritual beliefs.

What would others notice you doing that would tell them that you work from a Solution Focused approach?

I think people would notice a lack of negativity and experience greater empathy, and thereby feel welcomed in my presence in everyday interactions. People would also notice a difference in how personal and other matters are handled and resolved; in other words, not blaming people for things going wrong or not working out. They would feel more listened to and heard and feel respected in one's company, making it easier to relate and feel valued.

When women come into a shelter, they have been so busy surviving from one abusive action to another. The shelter is the first place of safety. A lot of women need to make a mental shift about domestic violence, as they tend to blame themselves: as one woman said, "My husband beats me because he loves me". I encourage women to tell their stories and then to rewrite them by not only reflecting on what was done to them but also focusing on the future. Just the mere fact that they are in the shelter means they have already started the process of change. Amplifying their courage to leave is vitally important, and I often ask, "What did it take to take the first step?" and "What enabled you to leave?" The shelter has even published a book written by 11 women who have survived abuse, and it is aptly titled *Rising up moving on* (Nisaa Institute for Women's Development [Nisaa], 2013). For me, the most powerful questions are about the future. They have left the violence and started the process of being safe, so inviting the future in is transforming. A shelter is your second most important decision – the first was to leave the danger and find the shelter. I help women to start thinking about tomorrow because the shelter is temporary. I encourage questions such as, "Where to from here?" and "What are your best hopes for your future?" The miracle question is one of the most powerful and valuable narrative changers and I always ask, "Suppose tomorrow your life is completely different because, remember, you have already left your past and taken a big step. What would you like to see happening differently tomorrow?"

Women who come from abusive relationships do not think about tomorrow. One woman even said, "I have never gone there, never thought about it". Another woman, Fikile Krolis (Nisaa, 2013, p. 115), wrote, "My bruises, pain, suffering and disappointment did not discourage me. In fact, it gave me the strength to go forward, work hard for the goals I want to achieve." I often encourage women to write a poem to reflect on their journey towards tomorrow. Writing down how you feel and what you think gives you an opportunity to reflect and move on. In 2016 we published another collection of stories written by teenage girls called *We are those girls* (Nisaa, 2016). Here is the poem written by Sharmim Meer (Nisaa, 2016) that inspired the title of our book and depicts how girls reframe, reflect, and take action to create a better future:

> *We are those girls*
> *Smiling through the storms*
> *Overcoming things thrown in our*
> *paths*
> *We are those girls*
> *Conquerors*
> *Beautiful, intelligent, wise, strong*
> *Proud of ourselves*
> *Willing to move forward*
> *Not judging or laughing at other*
> *Girls'*
> *wounds*
> *Sisters making a single bond*
> *Breaking the chain of fear*
> *Making our voices heard.*

Share an exercise that might be useful to other women practitioners

An exercise that is very helpful for women to build a bridge to the future and recognise their worth is the Circle technique developed by Arnoud Huibers and Ben Furman (2022). The Circle technique is an activity to help a client discover "resources, competencies and desired changes" (Huibers & Furman, 2022, p. 23). I have adapted the questions a little to suit our context and the clients we work with. The Circle technique is a simple activity that invites women to reflect upon their strengths and resilience, discuss and dream about a different future, and, on

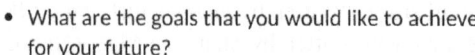

Outer Circle Questions:

- What do you want to change in your life going forward?
- What would you like to do differently from here on?
- What are the skills you want to learn moving forward with your independent life?

- What are the goals that you would like to achieve for your future?
- What are the lessons you can take from your past experiences?

Inner Circle Questions:

- What gives you hope about your life?
- What is the one way the world is better with you in it?
- What are you grateful for?
- In the next week, what is it that you can do to make your day special?
- In the midst of your difficulties, how do you manage to keep going?
- How have you coped so far?
- What are the little things that you are proud of?

Figure 17.1 The circle technique by Arnoud Huibers and Ben Furman

completion, gives the woman ideas on what to act on and how not to hold on to the ladder of her past, despite her pain. It is a drawing activity in which you invite the client to draw two concentric circles – the inner circle is to get to know the client and the outer circle is to discuss things the client wants to change.

I will illustrate how to use the exercise by sharing a case study. I have utilised and adapted some of these questions with a client from an abusive relationship.

My client is a 26-year-old woman who was in an abusive marriage for six months. She was emotionally and verbally abused by both her husband and her in-laws. She works at a bank and has a responsible job, which she handles well. She was referred to me because her ex-husband and his family do not allow her to live in peace even though they are divorced. I utilised questions from the Circle technique (Huibers & Furman, 2022) to help the young woman build a new life for herself.

The Outer circle questions are aimed at creating a future vision of possibility and a different tomorrow, and the Inner circle questions are aimed at reflecting upon strengths and resilience.

The questions were useful in the client's context and got her to think about her situation: where she wanted to be and what her goals were. She learnt to value herself and her contribution to her work and her family. The exercise helped her to gain emotional strength, start believing in herself again, and start thinking of a different life moving forward.

Share how you adapt the approach and make it your own. Give us five characteristics that are a part of your Solution Focused DNA

The five characteristics of my Solution Focused DNA are:

- I believe in and practice HOPE. Where there is life there is always hope. Hope and expectation lie at the core of my spiritual belief (Isgandarova, 2023) and my self-contentment and passion for being hopeful comes from being congruent with my beliefs.
- I firmly believe that life keeps changing and that everything is temporary. Despondency is temporary, pain is temporary, suffering is temporary, and we therefore can have a better tomorrow. Current experiences are not permanent. If we review the same experiences later, things will have changed. Hence change is the constant that accompanies us through life.
- I do not give up. I will never give up on empowering women and I will never give up on believing in women because I truly believe that the job I do is my life work, my calling, and I have never doubted that this is where I should be and what I want to be doing.
- My deep-seated belief is that if one solution does not work, another solution can always be found, instead of repeating the same problem-oriented mode and staying stuck. I also adhere to the philosophy that, "if it works, do more of it". When you are observant of your own worth, you can take another look at your life and ask, "What can I do differently?"

- Part of my DNA is to constantly work on myself and reflect on my development, my influence, and my spiritual growth. I have come to a realisation that as much as my clients need to work on their issues, I too need to ensure that I am constantly working on myself to become the best version of myself. Because I care deeply about women, I embrace my inner strength and potential to make a difference.

Which female practitioner inspires you and in which way?

I have been inspired by two women practitioners. The first one is Dr Jacqui von Cziffra-Bergs from Johannesburg, South Africa, who introduced me to the Solution Focused approach through the many webinars I was fortunate to attend. She is a great teacher and I have found the Solution Focused approach incredibly useful and have incorporated it into my repertoire of skills. I also appreciate the fact that Jacqui has a very progressive way of drawing me into further skills development. She frequently invites me or my organisation to new training with overseas Solution Focused experts. Her wanting to uplift Solution Focused practitioners is evident and appreciated.

The second practitioner who inspires me is Prof. Dr Nazila Isgandarova, who is an assistant professor at Emmanuel College at the University of Toronto, Canada. She teaches a programme offering Islamic Spiritual Care and Psychotherapy. She inspires me because of her work in incorporating an Islamic spiritual lens into Solution Focused Brief Therapy. According to Prof. Isgandarova (2023), not many people in the Muslim community seek treatment because of shame and guilt. In Islam it is believed that Allah (God) changes the condition of a person, when a person takes some sort of action to change and then places their trust in God (Isgandarova, 2023). This notion is very relevant, and I aspire to practise this myself and help my clients get there as well.

What soft small notion would you encourage other women practitioners to embrace?

We live in a world that is so divided and in which there is little tolerance for our differences as people, yet we have much in common as humans. I would encourage other women practitioners to embrace diversity and multiculturalism as a way of accepting all people who live on this earth. We know that small changes can lead to big results. Sometimes our own pejorative notions about groups of people cause us to distrust people, based on a lack of understanding of and clarity about others. If we, then, as therapists, have clients from other cultures and religions, our preconceived notions come into play in the therapeutic relationship and impact the outcome of the intervention. An example of one of my clients comes to mind. She is a Muslim woman who sought help from a therapist of a different race with a different value and belief system to her own. Because the therapist had the preconception of Muslim women being oppressed and uneducated, this became the therapist's initial perception of the client without even establishing rapport. The therapist assumed many untruths of her client without establishing the facts or clarifying and check-ing her understanding. The therapist was shocked during the sessions to learn that her client is, in fact, highly educated academically and spiritually, that she has a mind of her own, and expresses herself articulately, despite her dress code and her gentle disposition. The consequence was that the client quit therapy, as she experi-enced the therapist as patronising in her approach.

My best hopes for other Solution Focused practitioners

My best hopes for other Solution Focused voices are for this approach to be diver-sified among women of varying races, varying economic levels, and, in particular, from poorer communities who will benefit from this approach. Many women are deprived of psychotherapeutic help due to cost and accessibility factors. I believe that non-governmental organisations across the world can bring about transform-ation in society if they are trained in the Solution Focused approach. Women are crying out for help and in countries such as South Africa, where mental health services are far from accessible or affordable to the majority of the population, the Solution Focused approach can make a huge difference. If Solution Focused practitioners across the world came together as a think tank, solutions could be explored not only for South Africa but also for other needy regions where women do not have sufficient mental health services.

Since the Solution Focused approach is compatible with different value systems and spiritualities, it can assist and impact a wide spectrum of women. So, let's share our knowledge for the greater good and pay it forward. This is my hope for and challenge to the global Solution Focused community: let us make a transforma-tive contribution by donating and volunteering our time and let's start a Solution Focused mental health revolution for women now!

Co-constructive editors' reflection

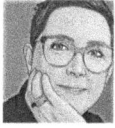

Zubeda is an interesting woman with an interesting story to tell. She brings in a different cultural and religious angle to our book and her context of working with women who have been abused is also very important. I think this is a very valuable chapter to add to our Solution Focused approach.

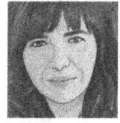

Being a Muslim woman in apartheid-era South Africa gave her firsthand experience of what it feels like to be disrespected and pushed aside.

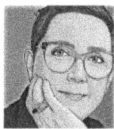

Zubeda's examples of her being mistreated and disrespected and how another woman stood up for her are strong examples of breaking pre-suppositions about women, and especially Muslim women.

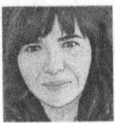

Yes, and what I found fascinating is on both occasions it was another woman encouraging her to share her voice, and this somehow gave her the resolve to never give up. I immediately thought of what Olga wrote about Insoo Kim Berg being like a pit bull terrier and not letting go and never giving up.

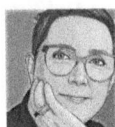

And this just makes me think of the chapters where it is clear that some of these women are on a very determined mission, you know, to achieve something. They want to make a change, not only in their own life but in the lives of other people as well. This is really, really powerful and strong. They have these really strong intentions to be helpful and create change.

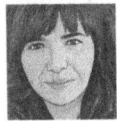

Yes, they want to make a difference and they will sacrifice a lot to make that difference.

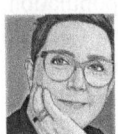

What I experienced when reading Zubeda's chapter, and her journey from the start to right now, was that it made me think that it is not one big step that gets you to where you want to be but rather several hundred steps that you have taken to reach where you are right now. And this leaves me full of respect and so impressed.

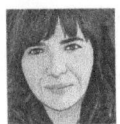

What stood out for me throughout the chapter was how her spiritual belief and her professional passion blend and flow together. Her spiritual belief of doing good is congruent with her professional values in everything she does.

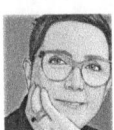

It is like a 3D picture; you know when all the components are put together you see the full picture. Zubeda stands on the Solution Focused assumptions and beliefs and they are similar to her religion or spirituality. And then what I was impressed by is how she started this women's shelter organisation. It's like, oh wow, she did it, and it has taken her a couple of years. She decided to support and help these women and their children because they have already taken the first difficult step by leaving. She wants to create a good environment for them now that they are already on their journey. And then she asks this beautiful question, "How can we support that journey further on?"

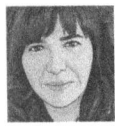

I love how she views the shelter as the second most healing step. The fact that they are at the shelter means that they have already taken the hardest step. This reminds me a little bit of those pre-session change questions, which assume that the healing has already started before meeting the person. The change started when a decision to do something different was made.

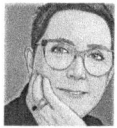

I can relate to that, and I agree because they have made the decision by themselves, you know, so there are pre-session changes that can be built on. This makes the descriptions into a preferred future so much more concrete.

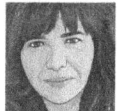

She's working on a presupposition that there is a preferred future already, just because you've already taken that step. And what I so loved is that she writes so beautifully how she finds the future-orientated questions the most helpful and the most important. She says it transforms people. And wasn't it interesting to read that a lot of these women have never even thought of a different future? But she goes back and keeps reminding them that it is possible.

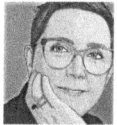

Exactly, and she keeps exploring their good reasons to leave. They have good reasons and they have decided to do this and just asking these questions makes the woman realise that she has done something good, decided something on her own, and she has decided that she already wants things to be different.

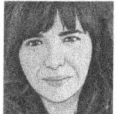

Yes, and she always invites a reflection, a reframe, and a possibility. And she does this by either doing an activity such as the Circle technique or by inviting them to write their stories. However, she invites them to write their stories with a better ending. These stories are not about the trauma but about what it took for them to get through it, to make a decision, and what the new ending looks like.

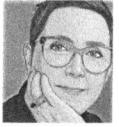

That is beautiful. And when she described her miracle question, she makes it a context marker, you know, because she reminds them, "You have already left your past and taken a big steps". She conceptualises the miracle question into the context in which they find themselves and focuses on the decisions that they have already made to create a better future. I really think that is brilliant.

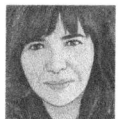

And then she invites them to write it down and, you know, a lot of these women have never, ever thought of writing their own stories. It is not in their repertoire, but she invites and encourages them to do so and then she celebrates their stories by even publishing a book.

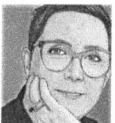

That is a strong signal of how important they are and how they have something valuable to share. Zubeda brings so much value into these women's lives. And to share it as a poem is so beautiful as well. "We are those girls, beautiful, intelligent, wise and strong. Proud of ourselves, willing to move forward" – it is such a strong message. And even though Julia wrote about Arnoud Huibers's Circle technique in her chapter, I think it is a great exercise for Zubeda to include because in the women's shelter it serves as a self-help tool.

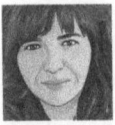

And then one thing Zubeda makes clear in her chapter is how much she works on herself. She's constantly on a self-reflecting mission. She believes that if she expects her clients to improve, then she too needs to improve and reflect on her own process.

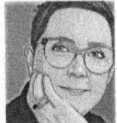

Yes, she is on a constant journey, which is part of her DNA. She has this belief in hope and she practises it as part of her spiritual belief. Another part of her DNA is this determination to never give up on empowering women. And the Solution Focused approach has given her a roadmap on how to empower and how to believe in them. This is inspiring because you can easily lean back and think, "Now I know what I need to know about the Solution Focused approach and about life". We can so easily become comfortable, and I think that she reminds all of us to be on our toes.

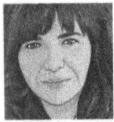

And then, Anne-Marie, I absolutely loved her best hopes of creating a Solution Focused revolution. A Solution Focused revolution on a multicultural level.

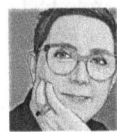

This is such a nice title, the Solution Focused revolution. I think that is a beautiful one.

Author references

Book, A. (2023). *The ripple effect of change*. Horizons UC Davies. https://humanservices.ucdavis.edu/news/ripple-effect-change#:~:text=%E2%80%9CI%20alone%20cannot%20change%20the,many%20ripples.%E2%80%9D%20%E2%80%93%20Mother%20Teresa

Equality Now. (2020, March 25). Gloria Steinem: 10 quotes from the frontlines for the fight for equality. https://www.equalitynow.org/news_and_insights/gloria_steinem_quotes/#:~:text=%E2%80%9CThe%20future%20depends%20entirely%20on,learn%2C%20but%20to%20unlearn.%E2%80%9D

Gouws, A. (2022, 2 December). Violence against women is staggeringly high in South Africa. *The Conversation*. https://www.news24.com/life/relationships/love/her_story/violence-against-women-is-staggeringly-high-in-south-africa-20221202

Ha, V.T. (2017, 29 September). World needs empowered women more than ever. *Vietnam News*. https://vietnamnews.vn/opinion/op-ed/394636/world-needs-empowered-women-more-than-ever.html

Huibers, A., & Furman, B. (2022). The Solution-Focused Circle technique: A visual tool for discovering strengths and facilitating change in therapy and counselling. *Journal of Solution Focused Practices*, 6(2), 6. https://doi.org/10.59874/001c.75018

Isgandarova, N. (2017). *Islamic counselling today: The case of domestic violence.* [Doctoral thesis, University of Toronto].

Isgandarova, N. (2023). *Solution Focused Brief Therapy from an Islamic lens.* [Video]. YouTube. https://www.youtube.com/watch?v=XaQbNIz46AY

Nisaa Institute for Women's Development. (2013). *Rising up moving on: Women writing our lives.* Nisaa Institute for Women's Development.

Nisaa Institute for Women's Development. (2016). *We are those girls: Writing our stories.* Nisaa Institute for Women's Development.

Chapter 18

Our Solution Focused revolution

Co-constructing our collective ideas

Anne-Marie Wulf (Denmark) and Jacqui von Cziffra-Bergs (South Africa)

Finally meeting each other

Reflections and co-constructions at Mabula Game Lodge, August 2023

This has been an incredible journey for the two of us; it has been life changing and life giving. After many Zoom meetings we finally met each other face to face here in Johannesburg, and the care and comradery was instant. Zoom really does create a connection; however, meeting in real life is so much better. What has been most surprising and even humbling is that, from the start, we have only received positive feedback, excitement, and encouragement from everyone we have contacted, spoken to, and invited into our book. Working on this book has created a strong sense of connection between stunning women doing amazing work – this project has enriched us personally as well as professionally, and has definitely enriched our Solution Focused knowledge as trainers. The flight around the world has left our Solution Focused passports full of incredible learning and, before we share our reflections, we would like to invite you to do this small reflective exercise to co-construct and build on your own learning.

We would like to invite you to reflect on your journey and think of what impressed you most. What stood out for you? What learning are you stamping into your Solution Focused passport?

- Reflect on the ideas you have gained, by travelling with the HopeCatcher, on a professional level. What are the golden nuggets?
- How has this journey been helpful to you in your work life?
- What ideas have you gained in terms of your own self-care?
- How have these stopovers expanded your vision on cultural diversity?
- What personal inspiration do you take home with you?
- What is the first small thing you are going to do in relation to your Solution Focused family, your network?
- How has this journey expanded your ideas on gender?
- Which small notion do you want to keep living by?

DOI: 10.4324/9781003430254-19

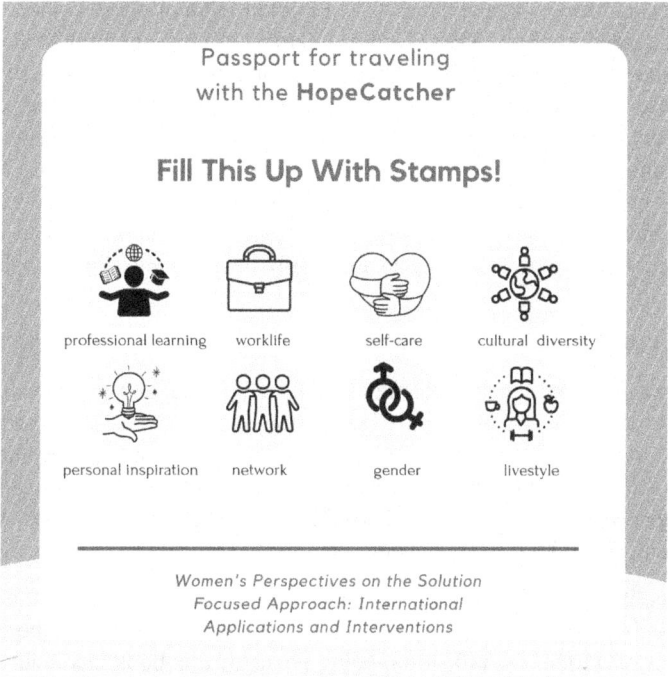

Figure 18.1 The HopeCatcher Passport

Write your own important learning in the stamps bellow:

Our Solution Focused passports filled up exponentially as we, the two editors of the book, sat down at Mabula Game Lodge and reflected on what we had learnt and what really stood out for us. We asked each other the following questions:

What impressed you about the book?

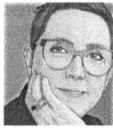

It is quite amazing to have reached what looks like the end of this project, and here we are sitting in a safari lodge reflecting on our journey. Saying this makes me think that, even though it is ending, there is something that will never end. We have formed a real connection with all the authors and a bond that I think will last forever. Women will keep on doing great Solution Focused work all over the world. We could easily have done a second edition with more unknown voices to be made known. These women are bringing so much hope, enthusiasm, and passion to their work. They are almost like activists in their fields working all on their own with strong beliefs and convictions. This book has shown us how the Solution Focused approach can be applied in so many different ways and in so many different contexts.

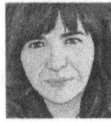

Yes, as I read the chapters I started thinking that all these authors are on a mission, they do not give up, and most of them are doing it alone. It has amazed me how powerful these unknown voices are. There are these incredible women doing incredible work with such determination and they are making a huge difference in the world. This really inspires me to not give up and to not only believe but also trust that my own little bit of good goes a long way. It is like a spiderweb that's constantly being spun, where each thread joins another thread and then you step back and see an amazingly beautiful interlinked web.

What impact did the book have on you?

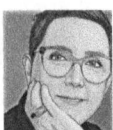

On a personal level I became even more humble, because I realised how many other women have been struggling on their own, spreading the word of the Solution Focused approach, as I have in Denmark. I feel so humbled and privileged that these women have given me a gift in their chapters, and I would love to go visit them, train with them, talk with them, just hang out.

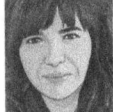

Yes, it has inspired me on so many levels, making me feel as though I am part of a community of women and not alone here at the bottom of Africa. On reflection, being a part of this book has made me more confident and given me permission to do the Solution Focused approach in my own way. I really feel that I belong to a group of incredible people, and it is as though their unknown voices have become a known reassurance in my head that I am not alone, that I can be creative, and that I can have my own personal style.

What surprised you about the book?

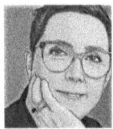

That nobody turned us down. Every person we asked to contribute gave a resounding "Yes". From the publishers to the endorsements to the foreword – and every single contributor. This really affected me and made me so joyful and happy. Whenever I shared the idea of the book with anybody, I always got, "Oh wow, that is such a good idea", which made me think this is our good reason for doing this book, because it is a good idea to share these unknown voices and it has made me so proud.

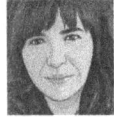

Yes, everybody loved the idea and I even heard things like, "It is about time that someone wrote about women in the Solution Focused field". Something that really bit me on the nose and surprised me was when we had just finished the first draft of Chapter 1 and that night, instead of feeling excited, I felt so uncomfortable. It suddenly dawned on me that the reason I was so uneasy was because all the references we had used in the draft chapter were from male Solution Focused authors. We both then went back to the drawing board, found all the books written by female practitioners, and rewrote the chapter. What really surprised me was how different the rewritten chapter turned out. Suddenly, there was a lot more emotional validation, more permission to be intuitive, and a lot more metaphoric language. The same Solution Focused concept of building a preferred future suddenly became a colourful journey incorporating all the senses, feelings, and dreams.

What difference did it make to you, reading these chapters?

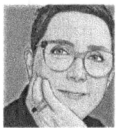

Making this platform of unknown voices heard has created a community of strong female practitioners and that has impacted me profoundly. I find myself speaking with a stronger voice and feeling really proud of being a woman. I realised there are so many women on a mission and it brings about so much hope. And this has been the golden thread through all the chapters, that we are all on a mission of bringing hope and resilience to the foreground, and supporting people in finding their preferred future.

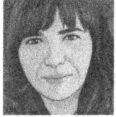

The realisation that compassion, kindness, and real empathy always comes first. I have always focused on the emotions my clients are feeling, I even explore them a little, contain and hold them, encourage them. However, I always felt a little guilty when I did that, like an imposter or a fake. After reading these chapters and meeting these amazing women, I no longer feel fake. Instead, I feel inspired and motivated to not only use my clients' feelings and incorporate how they feel but also give other practitioners permission not to shy away from emotions. Also, hearing how many of the authors integrate other approaches in the best interest of helping the client describe a preferred future has really empowered me to use everything I know, and by this I mean not only Solution Focused ideas. I have realised that it is all about being flexible and creative and integrating ideas into my Solution Focused questions, because ultimately it is about helping the client get to betterness.

What would others notice is different in your teaching and training of Solution Focused Brief Therapy?

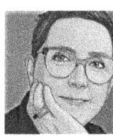

That I am less of a purist and more flexible in integrating things such as feelings and non-verbal expressions. It made so much sense to me when I read that there is a connection between the action and the feeling – not that I didn't know it, but I'd never thought of it in that way before. If we only look at and train the change and how it is shown in action and behaviour, we might be moving too fast. There is something between action and change, or that led to an action. There is something in-between: there's action, then a step back and pay attention to feeling, and then a focus on change and moving forward. More listening, more reflection, more allowing, and more perspectives.

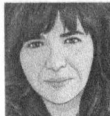 I believe I focus a lot on training people to listen with a Solution Focused ear and look with a Solution Focused lens; however, I want to do even more of it. I also want to help practitioners realise that all people have good reasons for doing what they are doing. The good reason is an attempt to solve the problem – maybe not always in a positive way, yet it is still an attempt at making life better or bearable. I also want to really concentrate on the idea of disruptive thinking and shifting the narrative. I have always taught people that Solution Focused questions create a pattern interruption and after reading these chapters I believe it even more – I would like to focus a little more on how we can not only disrupt the pattern but also create a new one.

What impact has being an editor and reading these chapters had on your practice?

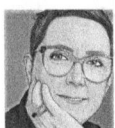 I am paying more attention to the non-verbal communication my clients show. I am also more creative and am definitely using more metaphors because I love metaphors and I want to use them more deliberately. Previously, I used metaphors by just improvising; now I want to be intentional with a metaphor. Also, I stick less to a fixed structure, and instead I go with my intuition. And reading all these amazing chapters, realising in how many contexts the Solution Focused approach works, made me think that the sky's the limit, there is no context in which we can't do Solution Focused work.

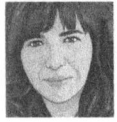 I have never liked labelling my clients and I am so humbled and excited to know that I am not alone in this. I am definitely going to listen to my inner voice even more and really go where it takes me in a session. I am also embracing my own style and my way of doing Solution Focused therapy a lot more. I have always played with language in sessions, but I am starting to teach my clients how to use language with more intention. As a resilience rebriefer, I have always woven my way back to resources, coping, managing, and signs of hope. What I want to do more of is learn how to step back and step back again when I get stuck, to really observe, slow it down, and wait for the resilience to show up.

What are the common factors that build our Solution Focused DNA?

As we reflected on all the common factors in each chapter, we realised that our Solution Focused DNA shows up in three main areas in our lives with an intersection between each. All the contributors mentioned that the Solution Focused approach influences their personal life, their professional life, and the way they interact in society. As we discussed these three main areas, we realised that there are definite intersections between each area and then a combined set of common factors found in all three areas.

Common factors on a personal level

From the chapters it became evident that all the authors use the Solution Focused approach as a life philosophy, as a way of being and living. It was thought-provoking that the Solution Focused way of **being** turned out to be an internal life coach, a way we speak to ourselves, a way we reflect on our lives, and a way we coach ourselves through life; almost as though we all end up having an internal Solution Focused coach who guides our language and helps our inner voices become Solution Focused and hopeful. What was also evident was the need to be authentic and true to yourself, value yourself, respect yourself, and use who you are to help others.

Common factors on a professional level

As Solution Focused practitioners we build relationships with people and not with the problem they bring. Because we all start from the same Solution Focused platform and search for our clients' desired outcomes, strengths, and hopes, we are all tailor-making our conversations to redirect our clients toward what they want and who they are. It's evident that we tailor-make conversations to lead the client from behind; we are all paying attention to not only the verbal but also the non-verbal; we are constantly building our conversations by relying on our gut feelings and thus creating our own personal style of **doing** the Solution Focused approach.

Common factors between the personal and professional level

For decades, attention has been paid to the relationship between the personal level of the therapist and the professional level, i.e., not becoming over-involved. However, it is unavoidable that we use ourselves, our knowledge, our intuition, and our emotions to help our clients to re-create not only their own lives but ours as well. This constant awareness leads to a co-construction of change where empathy and compassion are central and hope is given the opportunity to grow. And, as everything needs time to grow, the real skill lies in going slowly to grow fast.

Common factors on a society level

As we read the chapters, we realised all the contributors seemed to be on a mission. Of course, on different missions, as they work in different contexts, but skills such as focus, will, and determination are pervasive. They know what they want and where they want to go. We are all advocates of hope and of supporting people to manage and cope with their lives and create healthier societies. In order to be HopeCatchers we automatically place ourselves in a co-expert position using the resources in our society, focusing on the resources within our communities, and creating a culture of resilience building.

Common factors between the professional and societal level

As we advocate for resilience, using the community's resources and expertise, our conversations within our community always have a forward motion and future vision. Using the voices and ideas of all members of the community and considering each voice as valuable and worthy are a constant co-construction between people, a persistent co-partnership and cooperation between all involved toward betterness and change. As we co-construct and build a counter narrative, a counterbalance to the existing norm, we are elevating societal conversations with intentional hope language and a sense of possibility. This, ultimately, in our opinion, is ethical and just and builds towards social justice.

Common factors between the personal level and society

Being and **doing** Solution Focused transform us into activists for hope and change. The more Solution Focused we become, the more Solution Focused work we do, the more this creates a ripple effect of optimism and hope – not only within ourselves but also in our communities, encouraging partnerships of change and hope. When we are placed by society in a co-expert position, e.g. when doing an assessment of a prisoner, as a psychiatrist navigating medication, or within a legislative framework, our **being** and **doing** Solution Focused have a huge impact on a societal level.

What does our common Solution Focused DNA look like?

A resoundingly definite common factor of **being** and **doing** Solution Focused work in any **context** is that we are all HopeCatchers. This means that we all have a resilience, resource, and coping lens, and we look at everything through a lens of what is working, what is amazing, and what we can build upon. HopeCatchers lead from behind and sometimes from beside, using their gut feelings and intuition to empower people to visualise a better future. HopeCatchers build this vision of the future slowly, intentionally, and deliberately by being very selective in terms of

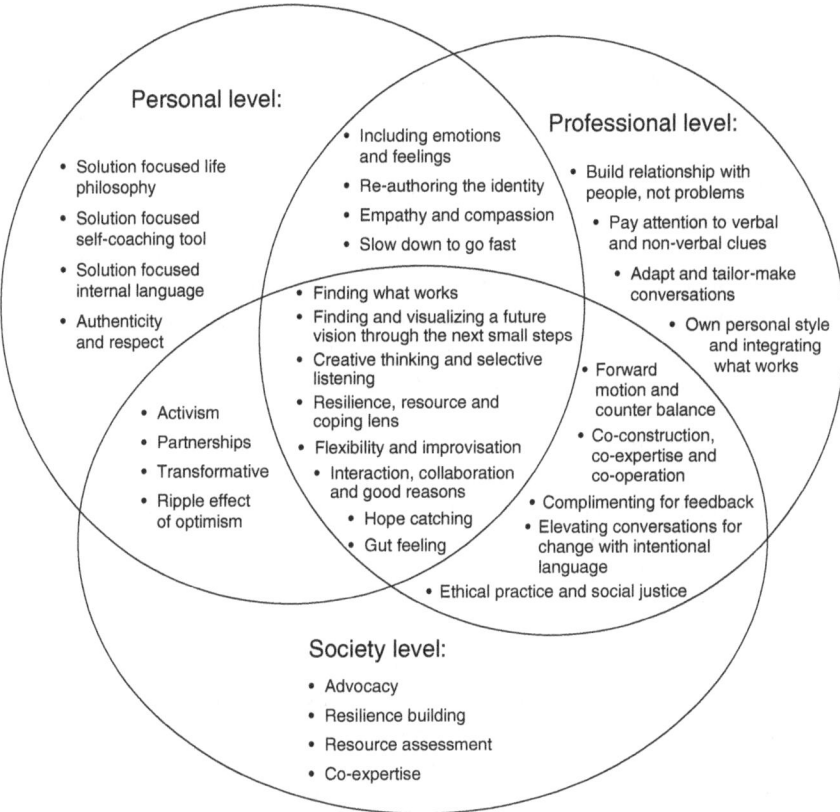

Figure 18.2 Three levels of common factors in our Solution Focused DNA

what they bring into the conversation and what they leave out, always with a good reason. As HopeCatchers we are all incredibly flexible and have the ability to adjust and improvise in the moment – in the best interest of our clients. HopeCatchers are collaborators and interact with clients to find the next small step to move towards betterness.

What are your best hopes for other practitioners?

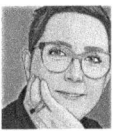

My best hope is that Solution Focused practitioners expose themselves to different trainers, see different Solution Focused DNAs, and, in doing so, discover their own DNA and their own unique way of being a Solution Focused practitioner. My best hope is that they are proud of themselves, of who they are becoming, and of what they are doing as a Solution Focused practitioner. I hope that they have the courage to stand up and use their own voices, talk from the heart, be transparent, and say what they wish for. If we do not express what we wish for, how will others know? Feelings, desires, and wishes need to be shown in interactions between people. Finally, I would love to see changes on a societal level, creating Solution Focused communities on larger scales.

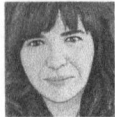

What really stood out for me about meeting more contributors is that we are all working with mental health, that we are all using the Solution Focused approach to make things better for people. My best hope is that we stay mindful of being in the business of betterness and hope and that we adapt the way we communicate to guide the conversations toward living life differently, more empowered, and more hopeful. My best hope is that we have fun in our work and see our clients as amazing people full of awesomeness. And, lastly, my best hope is that we use the Solution Focused approach in all aspects of our lives and spread it to as many people as possible so that we build people up and create positive change. Working in a Solution Focused way is such an adventure.

Summary

As we type our last words, we reflect on how the authors in this book have challenged us to look at our own presuppositions and assumptions regarding gender. We started our journey asking how our gender influences our work; however, we have realised that (perhaps) this question was embedded in an assumption that being a woman influences our practice. The authors have made us realise that gender exists on a continuum and is more fluid than ever. Our job is to be mindful of everyone's own, authentic self, regardless of gender. On reflection, the book has become a collection of beautiful Solution Focused exercises that can be used in so many different ways and contexts. This has been a true gift that each of us can apply and use in our practice.

Finally, it is also evident in all the chapters that we need to become and stay skilful detectors of hope. In each and every chapter there was this continuous mention of hope. Hope stands in the foreground and is our good reason for doing what we do. A Solution Focused mindset and practice provide hope by default. We are all on a worldwide mission of creating and maintaining hope, because without it there is nothing – and this is our Solution Focused revolution.

Contributors

Alesya Courtnage (she/her)

Alesya Courtnage received a Master of Arts degree from Drexel University, Philadelphia, in 2001 and has been practising as a psychotherapist in different mental health settings ever since. In 2008, Alesya attended her first workshop on the Solution Focused approach and fell in love with the hope, optimism, and respect that drive this way of working with others. Currently, Ontario is the epicentre of mental health walk-in clinics and her clinical work in this area inspired Alesya's interest in the potential of Single Session Therapy both as a service delivery model and as an effective clinical intervention. Within the past year alone she has provided training to over 1,000 front-line staff and continues to act as a consultant to many agencies across Ontario. Alesya is currently completing a PhD in Social Work.

Andrea Sandoval Riquelme (she/her)

Andrea Sandoval Riquelme is a clinical psychologist in Chile and has a master's degree in juridical psychology, a diploma in family mediation, and a diploma in the methodology of social investigation. With 20 years of experience dedicated to the practice of psychotherapy, she has worked at childhood protection non-governmental organisations with children, teenagers, and victims of child abuse, sexual abuse, and commercial sexual exploitation. She has also worked at a variety of universities, fulfilling management and teaching positions at undergraduate and postgraduate levels. She is currently practising as an independent clinical therapist while teaching at Centro Sol Institute, specialising in trauma. What she enjoys most about working with trauma patients is being able to witness people's ability to heal. She is also an amateur actress and stand-up comedian.

Anne-Marie Wulf (she/her)

Anne-Marie Wulf is a Solution Focused practitioner, trainer, and supervisor. She came across the Solution Focused approach in the late '90s as a social worker and lives and works in Copenhagen, Denmark. In 2016 she founded the Danish Solution Focused Institute offering a three-year training programme as Solution Focused Master Practitioner accredited by the International Alliance of Solution-Focused Teaching Institutes (IASTI). Today she mainly teaches, trains, and supervises. She is also the president of the European Brief Therapy Association (EBTA), a board member of IASTI, and an author of and contributor to several books. Anne-Marie differs depending on her context. With her grandchildren she is a playful, entertaining grandmother, and with her students she is someone who sometimes asks too many questions. No matter whom she is with, her life is rooted in Solution Focused assumptions about people.

Dragana Knezić (she/her)

Dragana Knezić was born in the former Yugoslavia and began working in Serbia after completing her psychology degree. Currently, she lives and works in Croatia and has mostly been working in non-governmental organisations as programme coordinator and human rights advocate. Dragana specialises in the rehabilitation of torture survivors and is known for her work with people on the move, with people living in poverty, and those in foster care. She also has a private counselling practice and works as an independent social policy researcher and expert.

Emma Burns (she/her)

Emma Burns has been a registered psychologist in New Zealand since 1996, working in mental health, education, traumatic incident response, family harm, and suicide prevention. Since 2010 she has been employed by the New Zealand Police, working with young offenders, families in harm, and, more recently, at an organisational level. The highlight of her career (so far!) has been developing a project called "Solution Focused Conversations in Custody". She also delivers free suicide prevention workshops for members of the public, has a small private counselling practice, and offers Solution Focused training to professionals and organisations. Emma is currently the president of the Australasian Solution Focused Association and is generally known as a mad advocate of the approach. Most importantly, she is a mother of four amazing young people, a competitive swimmer, and a chocolate enthusiast!

Hongyan Li (Julia) (she/her)

Hongyan Li is the co-founder of the Kids' Skills Promoting Center in China. She is also an advanced Solution Focused practitioner of IASTI. Julia, as she is fondly known, is the Chinese translator of a series of books about Kids' Skills (by Dr Ben Furman, 1998),
Respectful Parents, Respectful Kids (by Sura Hart and Victoria Kindle Hodson, 2006), and *Teach Like Finland* (by Timothy D. Walker, 2017). She worked in the

telecommunications industry for 30 years and entered the Solution Focused field at the age of 50. By teaching Kids' Skills in China, she allows ordinary parents and educators to benefit from Solution Focused ideas.

Jane Tuomola (she/her)

Dr Jane Tuomola has a private practice in Singapore where she has worked for over a decade. She works both as a clinical psychologist specialising in adult mental health and as a life and executive coach. She is a trainer, supervisor, and mentor coach at the Academy of Solution Focused Training in Singapore and SolutionsAcademy in Germany. Jane's particular area of expertise is supervision. She has been a clinical supervisor since 2006 and a coaching supervisor since 2018. She offers individual and group supervision, and teaches supervision coaching to therapists and coaches. She is interested in working cross-culturally and is co-editor of the book *Solution Focused Practice in Asia*.

Jacqui van de Velde (she/her)

Over the past 30 years Jacqui van de Velde has been working across the education, well-being, mental health, and community engagement fields in both a professional and a volunteer capacity in Australia, New Zealand, the European Union, Singapore, and North America. Jacqui is a trainer, speaker, and advocate for parent and family engagement, positive growth outcomes in education, professional learning networks and continuing education in the workplace, well-being, veteran health, and advocacy. Jacqui is on the board of two non-profits: Wellbeing Australia, a network bringing together people and organisations committed to developing healthy relationships that lead to individual and community well-being, and the Pro Patria Centre, a medical treatment and holistic care centre for veterans and first responders. Jacqui lives in the north of Sydney, Australia, is married to a fantastic man, and has two amazing children. At the time of writing she had just become a newly minted grandmother!

Jacqui von Cziffra-Bergs (she/her)

Dr Jacqui von Cziffra-Bergs is a practising psychologist from Johannesburg, South Africa, and teaches Solution Focused therapy and Solution Focused thinking to psychologists, social workers, schools, and organisations. Jacqui was an associate professor at the University of Johannesburg until 2013, when she left the university and started the Solution Focused Institute of South Africa. She still teaches at universities across the country on a consultancy basis and presents numerous workshops and webinars to her Solution Focused members throughout the year. Jacqui has written four books, with her last book for Oxford University Press entitled *Solution Focused Brief Therapy With Clients Managing Trauma*. She is married and has two sons who keep her feet firmly on the ground.

Katrin Berger (she/her)

Katrin M. Berger is married and has a son and two grown-up bonus sons. She lives near Bremen in Germany. As a qualified pedagogue, family therapist, and mediator, she works at a counselling centre for schools. She also works part-time as the owner of the "Lösungswerkstatt", where she offers Solution Focused training in addition to counselling and mediation. Katrin also coordinates networks for schoolworkers, both regionally and internationally. Occasionally, she also gives lectures or conducts workshops internationally.

María Amelia Barrera Morales (she/her)

María Amelia Barrera Morales is a psychologist in Chile, South America. She is a Solution Focused practitioner with the IASTI and the Denver Center for Solution-Focused Brief Therapy. María Amelia has been practising psychotherapy for 38 years and has taught at undergraduate and postgraduate levels. She is the founder of Centro Sol Instituto de Terapia Centrada en Soluciones Latinoamérica (Centro Sol Institute for Solution Focused Therapy in Latin America), where she has taught postgraduate courses, diploma programmes, and Solution Focused Brief Therapy courses since 2007. She participated in the book *Historias de cambio: El enfoque sistémico en acción* (*Stories of Change: The Systemic Approach in Action*, 2018), and co-authored the article *Implementación piloto del programa WOWW en una escuela privada en Chile* ("Pilot implementation of the WOWW programme in a private school in Chile", 2021). Her passion is to understand change and the strength of language and its resources.

Marie-Carmen Neipp (she/her)

Marie-Carmen Neipp holds a European doctorate in health psychology. She is a lecturer in the Department of Health Psychology at the Miguel Hernández University of Elche (UMH). Since 2015 she has also been the deputy Vice-Rector for Studies at the UMH. Marie-Carmen is a Solution Focused therapist recognised by the IASTI and a specialist in intervention and family therapy. Her research is mainly linked to the field of health psychology, focusing on the study of psychosocial variables and their influence on people's quality of life and well-being. In recent years she has also focused on researching the application of Solution Focused therapy and Positive Psychology techniques in different fields. She has participated as a researcher in various national and international projects and has more than 50 scientific publications to her name.

Olga Zotova (she/her)

Olga Zotova is a coach, psychotherapist, embodiment facilitator, and trainer from Moscow, Russia. In 2022 she moved to Tel Aviv, Israel, but she still works online with her Russian and international clients. Olga primarily works with adults on a variety of issues ranging from professional development and finding one's own path to more "therapeutic" themes, such as dealing with difficulties in relationships, handling crisis situations, and addressing past traumatic experiences. Regardless of the nature of a request, it is crucial for her to create a safe space that empowers people to connect to their strengths and values and move in their preferred direction. Olga's work is based on the principle of collaboration and she views life as a process where body, mind, and culture are interconnected. What helps her to stay hopeful despite the current political situation in her home country is her unwavering belief in people's resilience.

Rebekka Ouer (she/her)

Rebekka Ouer is a clinical social worker who specialises in Solution Focused work within the LGBTQ community. She owns and operates Dallas Rainbow Counseling, a private practice in Dallas, Texas, that has been serving this community since 2011. She has served as an adjunct professor at the University of Texas at Arlington's School of Social Work and is also a clinical supervisor for Licensed Master Social Workers in Texas. Rebekka frequently conducts training in Solution Focused Brief Therapy and the LGBTQ community and has authored a book for Routledge titled *Solution-Focused Brief Therapy with the LGBT Community: Creating Futures Through Hope and Resilience*.

Sofie Geisler (she/her)

Sofie Geisler is an adviser and international consultant on change strategies and processes, exponential action, and change narratives. She was among the first in the world to have introduced the Solution Focused approach in large-scale processes to governance and politics. With roots in Greenland and Denmark, Sofie is based in Mexico City, where she has worked in the public sector at federal, state, and local levels. She has a decade of experience using Solution Focus in the justice system, with special emphasis on alternative dispute resolution. Sofie has trained more than 1,000 lawyers, public servants, and decision makers in Solution Focused conflict and change management. She is currently working as a consultant in the Senate of the Republic of Mexico and as an independent adviser on political narrative and action.

Teri Pichot (she/her)

Teri Pichot, LCSW, LAC, MAC, has more than 30 years' experience working with some of the most challenging clients, including those who struggle with substance misuse, chronic mental illness, and domestic violence. She is the founder of the Denver Center for Solution-Focused Brief Therapy in the United States, and provides inspiring and educational training and workshops to professionals around the world on using this evidence-based approach with difficult clientele and within highly regulated, problem-focused settings. Teri has published numerous journal articles and five books (some of which have been translated into Spanish, Chinese, Japanese, Mandarin, and French). Learn more about Teri and her work at www. denversolutions.com.

Ursula Buehlmann (she/her)

Dr Ursula Buehlmann-Staehli, MD, FMH, is a specialist in child and youth psychiatry and a psychotherapist in Bern, Switzerland. Ursula has qualifications in Solution Focused Brief Therapy, Creative Children's Therapy, Hypnotherapy, and Traditional Chinese Medicine. She is a licensed supervisor, coach, and trainer, as well as the co-founder of creathera.ch. Ursula also serves on the board of the EBTA. See more at www.creathera.ch.

Zibeth Hansen (she/her)

Zibeth Hansen is a registered clinical psychologist who works with offender populations from a Solution Focused perspective. Her passion for the forensic field was fostered during her undergraduate studies when she majored in psychology and criminology. Her experience in the correctional setting started in 2008 when she was a camp facilitator and camp counsellor at @Risk youth camps for high-risk children. Zibeth has experience in a variety of correctional centres and with different types of offenders, including trial-awaiting detainees and sentenced offenders, and has worked in both medium- and maximum-security facilities. Zibeth has contributed book chapters detailing how she applies Solution Focused therapy in prison, appeared on a podcast discussing the work she does, and presented her work at several national and international conferences. She is currently employed in the Department of Correctional Services in South Africa and works primarily with male offenders in a maximum-security facility.

Zubeda Dangor (she/her)

Dr Zubeda Dangor is the founder and Executive Director of the Nisaa Institute for Women's Development. Zubeda is a clinical psychologist with a PhD in Psychology. Her PhD thesis has been published in a book entitled *Life After Abuse: An Exploration of Women's Strategies for Overcoming Abuse*. She received a postgraduate scholarship through the Institute of International Education to study at the University of Notre Dame in the United States. Zubeda was instrumental in initiating the National Shelter Movement and in establishing two shelters for women and children affected by gender-based violence. She served on the interim gender-based violence and femicide committee established by South African President Cyril Ramaphosa after the gender-based violence summit in 2018. In 2006, she received an international Community Service award from the organisation South African Women for Women based in Toronto, Canada. In 2015, she received the Woman of Wonder Award.

Index